Feline AIDS:

A Pet Owner's Guide

Feline AIDS:
A Pet Owner's Guide

By

Thomas Hapka

Published by Kitter-House Press, Whitewater, Wisconsin.

This book is NOT intended to replace veterinary care or any treatment regimen recommended by a medical professional. If your cat is experiencing health problems, seek professional help. Whenever possible, consult with medical veterinarians who also incorporate holistic treatment methods into their treatment strategies. The suggestions contained in this book were compiled from the personal experiences of the author and several medical and holistic practitioners. These recommendations are of a general nature and may not be suitable for your cat. Neither the author nor the publisher can be held liable for any adverse reactions to recipes, products or suggestions contained in this book.

Publishers Cataloging-In-Publication Data

Hapka, Thomas.
Feline AIDS : a pet owner's guide / by Thomas Hapka. --
Whitewater, Wis. :
Kitter-House, c2007.
p ; cm.
Includes bibliographical references.
ISBN 0-976458-0-1

1. Feline immunodeficiency virus infection--Alternative treatment. 2. Holistic veterinary medicine. 3. Cats--Diseases--Alternative treatment. 4. Cats--Health. I. Title.

SF986.I55 2007
636.8'089—dc22

LCCN: 2006903555

TABLE OF CONTENTS

This book is dedicated in memory of
JAC HAPKA (1980 – 1997)

ACKNOWLEDGEMENTS

To my family for their ongoing support. To Ray for his invaluable assistance in writing this book. To Barb for her steadfast support throughout the editing process. To Lita for her tireless work on behalf of animals. To the countless pet owners who strive to provide the best possible care for their cats.

In memory of Jac, Kitter, Garf, Lucy, Felix, Vinnie, Smokey, and the many other cats who brightened my family's home over the years.

INTRODUCTION

I would like to share the information my family obtained while caring for our own FIV+ cat. The information contained in this book was acquired from several medical as well as holistic vets, and our hands-on experience.

On June 10, 1995, our 15 year-old cat Jac was diagnosed with Feline AIDS. Jac was suffering from repeated upper respiratory infections, a loss of appetite, stiffening in his joints and subsequent difficulty walking, an overall loss of strength, severe loss of hair (it was coming out in chunks much like the hair of someone being treated for cancer), drainage from both eyes, and more. According to the doctor who did his blood-work, Jac was in grave condition and probably just a matter of days or weeks from death.

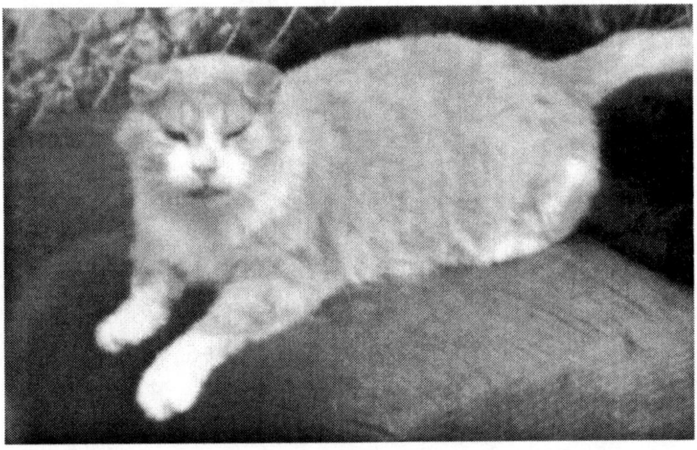

Jac, resting comfortably, one month after recovering from advanced FIV

At this stage in Jac's treatment, all medical options such as antibiotics and steroids had been exhausted. After an extensive search for information, my family learned about natural treatments for the first time. We introduced a combination of nutritional and homeopathic therapies to Jac's overall treatment strategy. He was able to recover from his immediate crisis and enjoy a high quality of life for the time he had left.

Jac passed away on November 11, 1997, of complications related to old age – not FIV. He was just a few months short of his 18th birthday. The vets who cared for Jac during his most critical phase were amazed that he was able to make such a dramatic recovery and enjoy a good quality of life for his final 2 1/2 years.

What follows is a summary of everything my family and I have learned through trial and error, as well as the information shared with us by the above-mentioned vets. By providing this information here, I hope to spare pet owners the frantic search for information we endured when Jac was initially diagnosed.

WHAT IS FELINE AIDS?

Feline AIDS, also known as the Feline Immunodeficiency Virus or FIV, is a feline disease that affects the immune system.

As the disease progresses, the immune system becomes impaired and the infected cat is left vulnerable to a variety of infections. Colds and otherwise routine infections can evolve into potentially life-threatening illnesses due to the absence of a normal immune system response.

Cats infected with FIV can remain free of symptoms for years. Once the immune system begins to degrade, however, symptoms emerge. Some common symptoms of FIV include:

- fatigue
- weight loss
- eye problems (runny drainage, and in some cases a gland resembling a third eyelid may cover a portion of one or both eyes)
- nasal congestion and reoccurring upper respiratory infections
- mouth problems (painful sores, bad teeth, irritated gums)
- dull, scraggly, or poorly groomed coat
- stiffening joints
- swollen lymph nodes
- diarrhea

Unlike other feline diseases, FIV is not wildly contagious. The primary means of transmission is through bite wounds during fights.

FIV has been found in both wild and domestic cats all over the world (from lions and tigers to typical American housecats). Scientists cannot conclusively determine how long this disease has existed. What should be noted is that FIV only affects cats. It is not a threat to humans.

There is no cure, but a diagnosis of FIV is not an automatic death sentence. With proper treatment, FIV+ cats can live for several years and enjoy a good quality of life.

The biggest obstacle faced by cats with FIV is late diagnosis. The onset of this disease is often slow and gradual. Pet owners typically fail to recognize the early symptoms.

In most cases, FIV is only diagnosed after the animal has lost weight, become weak, or developed a serious illness. Once the disease has been diagnosed, infected cats often suffer further injury at the hands of well-meaning medical vets who administer vaccinations, steroids, and other drugs that cause additional damage to the immune system.

The greatest successes in treating FIV have been enjoyed by practitioners using natural therapies. These treatment regimens typically involve comprehensive nutritional support through dietary improvements and vitamin supplements, homeopathic remedies, and the use of medications only as required. This is the approach I would recommend to any pet owner with an FIV+ cat.

GETTING STARTED

Cats with Feline AIDS have two fundamental problems:

- the disease is literally destroying their immune system;
- the disease robs infected cats of much needed vitamins, minerals, and proteins (a process that causes multiple health problems and accelerates the destruction of the immune system).

The best weapon to combat these problems is long-term nutritional support through foods and supplements. This important treatment option is frequently overlooked.

Medical vets who simply aren't aware of nutritional therapies often attempt to treat FIV+ cats with massive doses of antibiotics and steroids, as well as vaccinations. These are the worst things you can do for an FIV+ cat. In fact, such treatments can be fatal for a cat with advanced Feline AIDS.

I feel the need to make an important clarification. Drugs are sometimes necessary. Medications such as antibiotics can be quite useful WHEN THEY ARE USED PROPERLY. Unfortunately, these drugs are routinely misused.

In treating a cat with Feline AIDS, one cannot overstate the vital importance of nutrition. Cats infected with FIV require intensive nutritional support because the disease leaves them so depleted.

Dietary improvements and vitamin supplements can help to regenerate an ailing cat's immune system. Nutritional therapies are also effective as a preventative measure for FIV+ cats who are not yet showing symptoms. Any pet owner caring for a cat with FIV should begin with nutrition.

NUTRITION: A Powerful Weapon against FIV

Inadequate nutrition can weaken the immune system and lead to a variety of medical problems. Proper nutrition can help to boost and maintain the immune system, even in cats who are seriously ill.

Jac's condition improved after I modified his diet. In the first two weeks, he regained some of the weight he had lost, he became much more active and energetic, and his coat began to look shiny and healthy again. These results are not limited to Jac's case.

During the course of Jac's treatment for FIV, I consulted with three veterinarians who had medical as well as holistic training. Each of them used comprehensive nutrition to help keep FIV+ cats healthy, including many cats in the advanced stages of the disease.

Through my website on FIV, I have consulted in the rehab of hundreds of FIV+ cats. I regularly receive emails from pet owners who have seen improvements in their cats after increasing the nutrition in their diet. The degree of improvement varies from cat to cat, but the overall results from this approach are encouraging.

Working with FIV+ cats has taught me that proper nutrition is more than common sense. It is a powerful weapon.

Why Cat Food Isn't Enough

Now that I've emphasized the value of nutrition, I should explain what good nutrition is. The best way to start is by explaining what good nutrition isn't. Many pet owners believe they can meet their cat's nutritional needs with a bowl of wet or dry cat food. This is simply not true.

Keeping an FIV+ cat alive and healthy on nothing but cat food is difficult. Commercial brand cat foods like those sold in grocery stores are nutritionally deficient. They contain colorings and preservatives added by manufacturers to make the food more appealing to pet owners. These foods also have little real meat, and the meat they do contain is usually of poor quality.

Each year, tons of meat is condemned because of spoilage, bacterial contamination, or other impurities. This meat is not discarded. Instead, it is sold to pet food companies and used in cat foods that you see on your grocery store shelves.

Slaughterhouses are another major source of meat found in cat foods. When steak, chicken breast, and other prime cuts of meat are prepared for the public, there are leftovers. Lungs, intestines, and other indigestible parts, otherwise known as animal-by-products, are sold to pet food companies and used in cat food.

Even expensive cat foods like those sold by your vet DO NOT meet the nutritional needs of an FIV+ cat. These higher-priced foods don't contain adequate quantities of meat. The meat they do contain has been heavily processed and doesn't have much nutritional value. The bottom line is that there is no substitute for real meat.

Why Cats Need Real Meat

Just like their meat-eating relatives in the wild, cats need some real meat in their diet, especially raw meat, which contains an abundance of vitamins, minerals and enzymes. When meat is cooked, many of these vital nutritional components are lost. Serving your cats raw meat can be an effective way to provide them with a complete, natural source of nutrition.

I often receive emails from pet owners who are concerned their cat will get sick from eating raw meat. Unlike humans, cats are actually designed to eat raw meat. Before we came along, cats didn't kill a bird or mouse and throw it into the microwave for 5 minutes. They ate their food raw.

Over the past several decades, raw meat has been virtually eliminated from the feline diet as most pet owners have come to rely entirely on commercial brand cat foods. During that same period, immune system disorders, cancers and other conditions have emerged at epidemic levels. This is not a coincidence.

Medical research has shown that the elimination of raw meat from the feline diet is directly responsible for the sharp increase in feline diseases. Studies have further established that cats who are fed raw foods enjoy much better health than cats who eat only cooked foods. Arguably the most famous study on feline nutrition is commonly known as the Pottenger Cat Studies.

In this generational study, Dr. Pottenger used two groups of cats. The first group was fed a diet consisting of raw foods such as cod-liver oil, meat, bones, and milk. The second group of cats was fed the same foods, with one major difference. All foods served to the second group of cats were partially or completely cooked.

At the conclusion of the Pottenger Cat Studies, the cats in the first group were extremely healthy and did not require veterinary care. The cats in the second group, eating only cooked foods, developed health problems similar to those of today's American housecats (mouth problems, thyroid conditions, urological diseases, immune system impairments, and more). After three generations, the cats on the cooked-food diet were in steadily declining health, and they could no longer reproduce.[1]

The Pottenger Cat Studies clearly illustrate the importance of raw meat in the feline diet. Raw meat contains nutritional elements that help to support the feline immune system. In fact, many FIV+ cats improve once raw meat is added to their diet.

Safety Guidelines For Serving Raw Meat

In general, all raw meats are safe for cats. One notable exception is pork, which may transmit parasites if it isn't cooked prior to serving.

Common sense methods like hand washing and cleaning of kitchen surfaces and tools will keep you and family members safe from any risks associated with raw meats.

For the safety of your cat, purchase raw meats in small portions that can be used in a day or two. Discard any uneaten meats from your cat's dish within two hours. Be sure to thoroughly clean each dish with warm soap and water every day.

The Realities Of Feeding An FIV+ Cat

Cats are among the fussiest animals on the planet. Feeding a healthy cat can be a challenge because cats are so picky.

Feeding an ailing cat with FIV who doesn't feel well can be an even bigger challenge. It is critical to make the effort to find foods your FIV+ cat will eat.

If your cat has a food that he or she loves and will eat on a regular basis, don't take that food away in favor of an expensive food recommended by your vet. Most cats don't like so-called "veterinary grade" foods and subsequently won't eat them. Let your cat continue to eat his or her favorite foods, and offer additional, nutritionally rich foods.

When feeding a cat with FIV, there is one key rule to remember: KEEP YOUR CAT EATING AT ALL COSTS. If your cat will only eat chicken sandwiches from the local fast-food restaurant, that is far better than having him or her stop eating altogether. The best way to meet your cat's nutritional needs and keep him or her eating is through the use of an integrated diet consisting of dry cat food, wet cat food, and real meat.

The advantages of an integrated diet are logical. By offering your cat a wider variety of foods, you increase the chances that he or she will like something you are serving and eat. Integrated diets also provide far more comprehensive nutrition than diets consisting of just wet or dry cat food.

Feeding a diet consisting exclusively of dry food is not wise. Dry foods tend to be processed more than wet foods, and they have been linked to urological problems and kidney disease. Furthermore, not all cats can eat dry food.

FIV+ cats frequently suffer from mouth problems that make chewing painful. Cats with such mouth problems can literally starve to death in front of their food dish, unable to chew their food. Serving wet cat food assures that you are providing your cat with food he or she is capable of eating. Additionally, wet foods tend to be better sources of protein than dry food.

As I have already noted, real meat is an essential component of the feline diet. Boneless skinless chicken breast, chicken liver, fresh ground beef, and other raw meats can be excellent sources of nutrition for an FIV+ cat. Unfortunately, not all cats like raw meat. Furthermore, some cats have lost the ability to digest raw meat as the result of being fed nothing but commercial pet food.

For cats that don't like or cannot tolerate raw meat, you may have to serve lightly simmered meats instead. High quality cooked meat is still better than no meat at all.

How I Fed My Own FIV+ Cat

While my family and I were taking care of Jac, veterinarians recommended a number of foods to us. Some of these foods were suggested because of their immense nutritional value. Others are appetizers that can be helpful if your FIV+ cat isn't interested in eating. I will share some of Jac's favorites with you. You will need to experiment to find which foods your cat enjoys.

NOTE: In addition to the foods listed here, Jac also ate a variety of wet and dry commercial cat foods. At each meal, Jac received 9-Lives and Kozy Kitten canned cat food, Meow Mix dry food, whole milk, and a variety of raw meat.

RAW CHICKEN LIVER AND RAW SKINLESS CHICKEN BREAST: In their raw form, these foods have an extremely high nutritional content. Jac received these daily. Not all cats like these foods, but they are worth a try. I've heard from many pet owners who said their cats improved dramatically after they started eating raw chicken liver and raw skinless chicken breast. NOTE: Medical and holistic vets recommended these foods.

CHICKEN BROTH: You can cook a whole chicken or chicken parts to create homemade chicken broth. Allow the broth to cool before serving. If your cat won't eat, you can squirt the cooled broth down his or her throat in a syringe with the needle removed.

FRESH GROUND BEEF: At each meal, Jac received two to three tablespoons of raw fresh ground round or ground chuck. Raw beef contains valuable proteins and nutrients that can help to sustain a cat with FIV.

ALASKAN POLLOCK is a common fish found in most grocery stores. We cooked pollock for Jac in a frying pan, turning it often to prevent burning. It doesn't have the nutritional content of the above items, but many ailing cats will eat it.

WHOLE MILK is a good source of protein and calcium. Jac received fresh milk with every meal. We used whole milk whenever possible because it has a higher fat content and we were trying to help Jac maintain his weight. NOTE: It is a myth that ALL cats are sensitive to milk. Many cats have no problem digesting milk.

2 RAW SCRAMBLED EGGS in 1 cup of milk was another favorite of Jac's. Many cats will drink this mixture when they won't eat or drink anything else. NOTE: If your cat has never tolerated milk, this would not be a good idea.

LOW SODIUM, LOW FAT, SOLID WHITE TUNA IN SPRING WATER: Star Kist has developed this premium line of tuna that doesn't contain the salts and chemicals that otherwise make canned tuna a bad idea for cats.

DELI SANDWICH MEAT: Sandwich meat, sold at grocery store deli counters, can stimulate an ailing cat's appetite when nothing else appeals to them. Chicken breast was Jac's favorite.

BABY FOOD: Although baby food does not meet the nutritional needs of an FIV+ cat, its flavorful taste can get a sick animal eating again. This soft food is also useful for cats that have mouth problems. Chicken and beef were two of Jac's favorite flavors. NOTE: Be certain NOT to purchase baby food that contains onion, which is toxic to cats.

READY-TO-USE RAW FOODS: Several companies make raw food products, free of steroids, antibiotics, and other harmful substances found in some grocery store meats. These ready-to-use meals are convenient for pet owners, and they provide quality sources of protein for cats. The following are products I've had personal experience with.

Companion Natural Pet Foods, a Wisconsin-based company, makes premium quality raw foods for cats. Their web site is packed with useful information, including tips on how to safely introduce raw food to your cat's diet. (www.companionnaturalpetfood.com)

Primal Pet Foods, located in San Francisco, offers a variety of human grade raw foods for cats. (primalpetfoods.com)

VITAMINS

Vitamin supplements should be considered a MUST for any cat with Feline AIDS because these animals have such intense nutritional needs. Supplements are an effective way to address specific deficiencies and supply your FIV+ cat with more nutrition than food alone could provide.

Keep in mind that supplements are not a replacement for food-source nutrition. Nonetheless, vitamins are an important part of any FIV treatment regimen.

Creating A Feline Sports Drink

At the time of Jac's diagnosis, he was very ill, and medications had stopped being effective. There was no commercially available vitamin product for cats with FIV. Jac's condition was obviously getting worse, and I had to get innovative in order to provide him with the vitamins he needed.

Working with a number of medical and holistic vets, I came up with a feline "sports drink" of sorts. It contained the vitamins that Jac's doctors felt he needed most. While caring for Jac, I made several different versions of this drink. I'll provide you with the recipe I still use when caring for FIV+ cats.

Simplified Version Of Jac Hapka's Sports Drink	
Vitamin C (Mega C, calcium ascorbate, or Ester C)	8,000 mg
Vitamin E (400 i.u. softgels)	6 capsules
Vitamin A (10,000 i.u. softgels)	6 capsules
Acidophilus (powder or capsules)	The highest potency you can find
Calcium (see product index)	250 mg
Brewer's Yeast powder	3 tablespoons
Pycnogenol	3 capsules

I rarely purchase vitamins at pet stores. Supplements made for animals are often of poor quality, and they typically contain doses of vitamins that are too small to have a health benefit. There are notable exceptions.

Mega C and the Animal Essentials product line, for example, are high quality supplements specifically designed for cats. Many holistic practitioners use and recommend these products.

Although the feline sports drink calls for brewers yeast, I sometimes use B-complex vitamins instead. Some cats are allergic or sensitive to brewers yeast, and may develop itchy, irritated skin while receiving the supplement. For these animals, B-vitamins are a necessary substitution.

It's important to note that B-complex supplements designed for humans are not suitable for cats. They are extremely bitter – enough to make many cats choke or vomit. If you decide to use B-complex vitamins in the sports drink, use a supplement that is designed for cats.

Most of the ingredients in the sports drink are supplements made for humans. Health food stores are generally the best source for quality supplements. Their products contain the fewest fillers, flavorings, and preservatives. This is important because these unnecessary ingredients can make a supplement less digestible.

All of the ingredients in Jac's sports drink can be mixed in the blender with 1 cup of water and at least 3 scoops of Häagen-Dazs or Breyer's vanilla ice cream (these brands have the fewest binders, colorings, and preservatives). It usually takes 3 to 5 minutes to break these down into a liquefied state. If the mixture appears too thick, I add a little water.

If your cat doesn't drink milk you can leave out the ice cream and mix all of this in water (but it will taste horrible). Another option is to purchase a container of the milk substitute that so many vet clinics and pet stores carry. It helps with the taste problem and gives the drink a better overall consistency.

Initially we gave Jac 6 cc's of this drink four times per day. We simply squirted it down his throat in a syringe with the needle removed. However, each animal is different. If you choose to try this approach, you may want to begin slowly – 3 cc's once per day is a good place to start. See how your cat tolerates it before going further.

Your cat may reach his or her bowel tolerance (the point where gas, loose stools and diarrhea begin, at which time you slightly reduce the amount of Vitamin C until stools are a little better formed and gas is reduced).

When administering the drink, aim toward the back of the mouth and off to either side. If you squirt down the middle of the cat's throat, some of the drink could get into the lungs. Direct any questions to your veterinarian (they administer oral medications every day).

Alternatives To Force Feeding Vitamins

Not all cats are suited for having meds squirted down their throat. Some animals find this process quite traumatic. Wrestling FIV+ cats to the floor and forcing vitamins down their throat is unwise. At that point, the stress of the process far outweighs any benefit provided by the supplements. For these cats, Jac's sports drink won't work and an alternative is required.

There are two products that work well for cats who can't handle having vitamins administered forcibly. I mix these powdered supplements with a small amount of flavorful food I know the cat will eat (usually a teaspoonful of baby food or canned cat food with lots of gravy to it).

NOTE: You should NOT taint all of your cat's food with vitamins. Some cats will not touch their food once supplements have been added. You don't want your cat stop eating because all of his or her food is tainted with strange-tasting supplements.

Mega C: This premium vitamin C supplement is used by many holistic practitioners to treat cats with viral infections and immune system disorders. It contains a blend of vitamins and minerals, including vitamins A and E. The product has a bitter taste that some cats don't care for. However, Mega C is highly concentrated, so only a small amount of the supplement is required. Just mix a pinch of Mega C powder into a flavorful moist cat food.

BioPreparation, manufactured by BioNutrition (www.biopreparation.us), is a potent natural supplement derived from algae. This remarkable product is nutritionally rich, containing an abundance of enzymes and more than 5,000 naturally occurring nutrients, including vitamins, minerals, essential fatty acids, and complete proteins with more than 20 amino acids. BioPreparation also has immune boosting properties that can benefit animals with a variety of medical conditions. Holistic practitioners administering this product have reported dramatic improvements in cats afflicted with cancer, including substantial tumor reduction. There are two BioPreparation formulas. F2 is intended for general support and preventative applications. F3 is a more intense formulation used for advanced conditions such as cancer. Some practitioners recommend starting slowly, initially using just a pinch per day of the F2 formula and increasing gradually. BioPreparation is not a substitute for homeopathy and other natural therapies, but it can be an invaluable addition to your cat's FIV treatment regimen.

HOMEOPATHY

Cats with FIV routinely develop medical problems that nutrition alone cannot resolve. My own FIV+ cat experienced three serious medical crises that nearly claimed his life. In circumstances like these, where the medical community can offer no help and nutrition isn't enough, homeopathy can be very useful.

Homeopathy has proven remarkably effective in treating so-called "untreatable" conditions like liver disease, kidney disease, and FIV. The practice of homeopathy can be difficult to explain because it is based on such a unique set of principles. Many people confuse homeopathy with herbalism. For purposes of clarification, homeopathic remedies and herbal remedies are not the same thing, and they function in very different ways.

In homeopathy, substances that produce certain symptoms in a healthy person are used to cure a patient suffering from those same symptoms. For example, a substance that would cause high blood pressure in a healthy person might be used to treat a patient suffering from high blood pressure. It is not exactly clear how this process works, but holistic practitioners believe that homeopathic remedies somehow stimulate the immune system and enable the body to heal itself.

Homeopathic Doses

Homeopathic doses are quite different from those of mainstream pharmaceuticals. With prescription and non-prescription drugs, higher doses are more powerful. The larger the dose of the drug, the more powerful the result. In homeopathy, the reverse is true.

Homeopathy is based on the principle of the minimum dose. Homeopathic remedies are made from a natural substance which is then diluted by 1 part to 1,000, 1 part to 1 million… even 1 part to 1 billion. The greater the dilution, the more powerful the remedy is.[2]

The dramatic recoveries experienced by critically ill animals receiving homeopathic treatment clearly show that it does work. Scientists, however, cannot explain how such diluted remedies can have any health benefit. The answer may lie in the process by which remedies are made.

During the process of making a homeopathic remedy, an original substance is diluted and thoroughly shaken. Sometimes these substances are shaken several thousand times. Homeopaths believe this process of diluting and shaking releases the energy of the original substance. Since it is the energy that promotes healing, remedies can still be very effective even when diluted to the point where there are no molecules of the original substance left.

Choosing The Right Remedy

Prescription and non-prescription drugs tend to be used in a "one size fits all" manner. By stark contrast, homeopathy is a highly individualized practice. Because homeopathy is so individualized, it is not uncommon for cats with the same disease to be treated with completely different remedies.

Selecting the right remedy is essential to effective homeopathic treatment. Homeopathic practitioners choose the correct remedy for a patient by evaluating the individual's symptoms. The symptoms of the patient must match up well with the symptoms associated with the homeopathic remedy.

If the patient's symptoms and the remedy selected do not match up well, a cure will not be achieved.

Potency is another important factor in selecting a remedy. Lower potency remedies such as 3X or 9C are milder than higher potency remedies like 200C or 1M. As a result, they are less likely to seriously aggravate the patient's symptoms.

Administering Remedies

Another unique factor of homeopathy is that remedies require special handling. They can be neutralized and rendered ineffective by excessive heat, sunlight, and strong smells like camphor and eucalyptus. It is also important not to handle homeopathic remedies.

The ideal method of administering remedies is to drop them directly into the cat's mouth. For cats who don't cope well with receiving oral medications, hide a remedy in a small amount of food. Flavorful canned foods with lots of gravy seem to work best. Remedies have no taste or smell and usually dissolve quite well in a teaspoon of moist cat food.

Skepticism About Homeopathy

There are two centuries of clinical evidence to show that homeopathy does work. It has been used to treat humans and animals all over the world. Against FIV, homeopathy has proven highly effective. Despite this fact, many people are still skeptical of homeopathy. Much of this skepticism comes from the fact that it cannot be scientifically proven.

There is no medical device or laboratory test that can measure the energy on which homeopathic remedies are based. As a result, it is not possible to produce the type of hard, scientific evidence that would satisfy the medical and scientific communities.

I must admit that I was skeptical about homeopathy when it was first presented to me. The whole concept that these diluted remedies containing "energy" would somehow help my cat seemed like witchcraft. My opinion didn't change until I had the chance to see homeopathy work firsthand.

Jac was seriously ill, and nutrition alone wasn't enough to keep him healthy anymore. Blood tests revealed that Jac's immune system was failing and he was fighting a serious infection. All of the doctors I consulted agreed there was no medical treatment available for Jac's condition, nothing could be done, and they expected him to die in a matter of days. Since I had absolutely nothing to lose, I decided to give homeopathy a try. The results were amazing.

In less than a week, Jac regained some of his strength, and his upper respiratory infection began to clear. He even made attempts to play with our younger cats. Follow-up blood tests revealed dramatic improvements in Jac's condition. Any doubts I had about the effectiveness of homeopathy were now gone.

Jac's incredible recovery is not an isolated case. Every day, holistic practitioners use remedies to treat FIV+ cats for a wide range of problems. This approach consistently achieves positive results. I would urge those of you caring for FIV+ cats to put aside any skepticism you may have and include homeopathy in your treatment strategy.

When To Consult A Doctor

Before embarking on any homeopathic regimen, it is essential to make sure that you actually know what your cat's medical problem is. Otherwise, you could inadvertently treat your cat for the wrong condition. This is where a consultation with an experienced medical vet can be useful.

Diagnoses of FIV, liver disease, and kidney disease, for example, can only be verified through blood tests. Obtaining a formal diagnosis of your cat's medical problems will help to assure that you select the correct homeopathic remedy. If you have already begun treating your cat homeopathically and the animal isn't responding, a medical consultation is a wise precaution.

Some medical problems, such as acute illness or injury, require medical intervention. Locating fractures or bowel obstructions can only be done with x-rays. Severely dehydrated cats often require IV fluids. Removing obstructions from the throat or repairing large wounds generally requires surgery. These are examples of a few problems that cannot be treated with homeopathy alone.

Whenever possible, I recommend using a veterinarian who has medical as well as holistic training. Without fail, doctors trained in both disciplines have the finest diagnostic skills. They also have the added advantage of being able to treat your cat medically or homeopathically in any circumstance. If you don't have such a vet in your area, work with your local vet for acute diagnoses, and do a phone consultation with a holistic vet to choreograph your cat's overall treatment strategy.

Understanding The Process Of Homeopathic Consultation

In a conventional medical consultation, cats are often rushed into and out of the vet's office in a matter of just a few minutes. Diagnoses are made quickly, and with minimal information. Symptoms are then treated with prescription or non-prescription drugs.

The primary drawback of this symptomatic approach is that it doesn't truly resolve the problem. Medications temporarily mask the patient's symptoms, and once the drugs wear off, the problem returns. Since the root cause of the illness is not being addressed, the patient never truly recovers, and repeated symptomatic treatment is required.

A few months ago, I corresponded with a woman from Texas who had taken her cat to the vet more than ten times for skin irritation. Each time, the vet treated the problem with steroids, antibiotics, and skin creams. This would relieve the irritation for a matter of days, but the problem would return. After several weeks and hundreds of dollars in vet bills, it turned out the cat was allergic to an ingredient in his food, and that was causing the skin irritation. This is a perfect example of how a strictly symptomatic approach can fail to resolve a medical problem.

Homeopathic practitioners understand that symptoms are the result of an underlying illness or condition. Instead of merely suppressing symptoms, they attempt to determine the root cause of the patient's illness and select the right remedy to resolve the problem. To accomplish this, homeopathic practitioners need to know as much as possible about their patients.

In a typical consultation, the practitioner will want to discuss more than just the acute symptoms that prompted you to make an appointment. You will most likely be asked to describe any changes in your cat's diet, appetite, behavior, or activity level. The practitioner will also want any available details about your cat's medical history (surgeries, major illnesses, vaccinations, and so on). This may seem like a great deal of information to provide, but it is necessary.

Each homeopathic remedy has a list of physical and emotional symptoms associated with it. The homeopathic practitioner must choose the remedy that matches up best with your cat's symptoms. The closer the match, the better the result. By providing the best possible information about your cat, you can increase the chance that this optimum remedy match will be achieved.

COMBINATION REMEDIES: Another Approach To Homeopathy

Classical homeopathy is based on the principle of finding one remedy that matches up with a cat's symptoms. This approach is effective in treating medical problems that only involve a single organ. For conditions like FIV, which attack multiple systems of the body simultaneously, combination remedies are often more effective.

Combination remedies are sometimes referred to as shotgun remedies because they take a broad-spectrum approach to homeopathic treatment. Finding the ideal remedy for any specific patient or condition can be profoundly difficult and time consuming. I've seen highly skilled practitioners struggle to find the right remedy, especially when treating cats with complicated conditions.

Combination homeopathy attempts to bypass this often frustrating selection process by incorporating several remedies appropriate for a given condition, hoping that one or more of them will produce a recovery. For example, a combination remedy for nasal congestion might contain as many as fourteen different remedies. Some of these might be remedies that stimulate the immune system, while others could be remedies commonly used for decongesting the sinuses.

Combination remedies are becoming increasingly popular tools in the treatment of diseases like FIV. Such diseases often cause too many problems for a single remedy to address. A good combination remedy, however, can fight infection, stimulate the immune system, combat fatigue, flush toxins from the body, and perform numerous other functions at the same time.

Effectiveness aside, there are also economic realities to classical homeopathy. The price of a single homeopathic consultation is comparable to that of a comprehensive medical appointment. Ongoing treatment, however, can become very expensive.

While I was writing this book, my sister consulted a holistic practitioner when her newly adopted kitten became seriously ill. The animal's condition was complex, and multiple telephone consultations were required daily. In less than two weeks, the bill came to one thousand dollars.

I've heard from devoted pet owners who desperately wanted to help their FIV+ cats but simply couldn't afford the hourly rates of a classical homeopath. For such individuals, combination remedies provide an affordable, user-friendly alternative.

Combination remedies eliminate the need for the painstaking remedy selection process. If the label on a combination remedy reads "Liver Disease", that's exactly what it treats. Because they are easy to use, these remedies make homeopathy accessible to pet owners.

HERBALISM AND HERBAL REMEDIES

Some holistic practitioners use herbal remedies in the treatment of FIV. Although I believe that many herbal products offer a substantial health benefit, I generally prefer to see them selected and administered by a trained professional.

Herbal remedies can produce side effects like nausea and stomach upset. Serious reactions can occur if excessive doses or inappropriate combinations of remedies are administered.

My own cat had an adverse reaction to an herbal remedy, but fortunately, it wasn't serious. I purchased an herbal echinacea tincture recommended in a cat book for boosting the immune system. The moment this product hit Jac's tongue, he began flailing his head, and profusely thick mucous poured from his mouth. Fortunately, he recovered in a matter of minutes.

The next day, I consulted with a holistic practitioner who explained that what happened to Jac is not uncommon. Cats have extremely sensitive mouths. Many herbs have a strong taste that can irritate a cat's mouth, causing the type of profuse salivation and choking that Jac experienced. This is one drawback of herbal therapy.

Finding a way to administer herbal products safely can be a challenge. Forcing herbs down a cat's throat can cause severe irritation or choking. Placing herbs in a cat's food is equally unwise because the animal might still choke or simply stop eating.

FIV+ cats can benefit from herbal remedies. However, because of the potential risks, I usually won't administer these products without the guidance of an experienced holistic practitioner. There are exceptions, however. The following products are safe, effective, and buffered with glycerin to reduce the risk of choking or stomach upset.

Ashwaganda, made by Ayush Herbs (800.925.1371), is a potent herb often used to rejuvenate ailing cats. I credit this product with saving two of my own FIV+ cats who were weak, anemic, and appeared to be dying.

Herb Pharm (http://www.herb-pharm.com/) makes an alcohol free, glycerin based Golden Echinacea tincture. Some practitioners recommend 3 drops twice per day for one or two weeks to help resolve stubborn infections.

Animals Apawthecary (animalessentials.com) has developed a premium line of user-friendly herbal tinctures for a broad range of conditions.

If you choose herbal remedies for your cat, proceed cautiously. Start with very small doses, and watch for signs of adverse reactions. Don't attempt to mix your own combination remedies. Use commercially prepared products like those I've listed here. They've been carefully formulated by skilled professionals to reduce the risk of choking or serious reactions.

Whenever possible, consult an experienced practitioner who can determine which remedies are appropriate for your cat.

CHIROPRACTIC CARE

Chiropractic adjustments have become an increasingly popular form of natural treatment for cats in recent years. Many pet owners don't realize there are some potentially serious risks to chiropractic treatment.

Any time that bones in the neck and spine are manipulated, especially when the technique is applied with too much speed or force, veins, blood vessels, and nerve endings can be damaged or even severed. When this occurs, the results are devastating and may include brain damage, pain, or paralysis. I know about this type of injury from personal experience.

In July of 2000, I went to a chiropractor for what was supposed to be a routine adjustment. The chiropractor relaxed the muscles in my neck with a series of massage techniques. Once my neck was completely limp, he whipped my head to the left with a quick, jerking motion. This technique is known as a high velocity adjustment, and it is a common practice in chiropractic care for humans as well as animals.

As soon as my neck was manipulated, my eyes began to rotate in the sockets and I felt as though the earth were spinning at 300 miles per hour. From the chiropractor's office, I was transported to a hospital, and I nearly died as the result of brain damage. To this day, I am still recovering from the physical and psychological affects of my chiropractic injury.

I was later informed that the chiropractor had torn my vertebral artery, one of the major arteries that deliver blood to the brain. The end result was a bow hunter's stroke, a form of brain injury that results when the neck is placed at an extreme angle while under pressure. This injury is so named because it is often seen in bow hunters. Each year, growing numbers of people are suffering bow hunter's strokes as the result of chiropractic treatment. I am sorry to report that at least some animals have been injured in this fashion as well. What happened to me could easily happen to your cat.

Although my family has seen the damage chiropractic care can cause, we have also reaped its benefits. One of our cats, Blackie, would not be alive today if it hadn't been for the work of a skilled chiropractor.

In 1994, Blackie was born in my parents' garage when a wild stray wandered in and gave birth in a basket near my father's workbench. At the age of four weeks, Blackie learned how to climb. On a Wednesday afternoon, she climbed several feet above my father's workbench, and fell to the concrete floor of the garage. I heard the impact and came running to find that Blackie was alive, but her head was upside down. The impact had literally jammed her neck and rotated her head 180 degrees.

I rushed Blackie to the local vet clinic for emergency treatment. The doctors there were stunned, and they explained to me that kittens are very flexible. If Blackie had suffered that same injury as an adult, she would have likely broken her neck and died upon impact. Either that or she would have been paralyzed.

For almost two hours, puzzled medical doctors examined Blackie, trying to figure out some way of treating her injury. They placed calls to several veterinary schools, and I was told the only option was a dangerous surgical procedure that would most likely kill Blackie or leave her permanently disabled. Obviously this was not a reasonable course of treatment, and I made a few phone calls of my own.

In a nearby town, I found a chiropractor who specialized in treating cats. She spoke with the doctors and urged them to give Blackie some muscle relaxants and anti-inflammatory drugs to keep her neck from swelling and stiffening. She also asked for a complete set of detailed x-rays so she could study the anatomy of Blackie's neck. The doctors were skeptical about working with a chiropractor, but they complied.

Over the course of the next five days, the chiropractor administered a series of gentle adjustments to Blackie's neck. With each day, her head came closer and closer to its original position. By the following week, Blackie's head was back in its normal position, and she is now a very healthy, active adult. In Blackie's case, chiropractic care proved to be a lifesaver.

Due to the risks involved, I prefer to reserve chiropractic care for cases like Blackie's where there is a mechanical injury, and the medical community has no safe treatment to offer. I never use chiropractic care to stimulate the immune system in FIV+ cats because there are much safer, equally reliable ways of accomplishing that.

I have found that experienced massage therapists can stimulate the immune system and relieve pain in FIV+ cats, without the risks involved with chiropractic care. I would urge any pet owner to pursue this gentler, safer option before ever considering chiropractic care. If you choose chiropractic care for your cat, there are some important guidelines to follow.

Chiropractors who aren't trained to work on animals often make the mistake of applying the same physical force to a cat that they would apply to a human being. This can result in serious, possibly permanent injury. Cats have far more delicate anatomy than we do, and they require a gentler touch. Always make sure that you are working with someone who has extensive experience in treating cats.

Furthermore, do not allow your cat to be subjected to high velocity adjustments. These techniques are by far the most likely to cause injury. Work only with a practitioner who uses low speed, low impact manipulations. This can greatly reduce the risk of injury.

Lastly, diseases like FIP (Feline Infectious Peritonitis) can drastically weaken the walls of blood vessels, arteries and veins, potentially leaving a cat more susceptible to chiropractic injury.

Before embarking on a chiropractic regimen, work with a good vet to make absolutely certain that your cat does not have any conditions that would leave him or her predisposed to chiropractic injury.

FREQUENTLY MISUED MEDICATIONS

Natural treatments are the focus of this book. Proper nutrition, vitamin supplements, and homeopathy are essential to any cat with FIV. There are, however, occasions when prescription and non-prescription drugs are necessary. I often encourage pet owners to seek medical assistance for their cats. My own cats receive regular medical exams, and they have occasionally been treated with drugs prescribed by our local vet.

When used properly, medications can be beneficial. Unfortunately, some medications are frequently misused in the treatment of Feline AIDS. In some cases, the consequences can be serious. My goal is to spare FIV+ cats these inappropriate treatments.

ANTIBIOTICS

Because of their impaired immune systems, FIV+ cats frequently develop secondary infections, such as respiratory and sinus infections. In most cases, these infections can be treated naturally, especially with the help of an experienced holistic professional. However, antibiotics are sometimes necessary to resolve stubborn infections that won't respond to natural treatments.

When used properly, antibiotics can stop an infection from going unchecked and evolving into a more serious illness. Unfortunately, antibiotics are often used inappropriately, especially in the treatment of FIV.

Many medical vets prescribe long-term courses of antibiotics for FIV+ cats as a preventative measure. In fact, some doctors place cats on antibiotics the moment they test FIV+, even if the animals have no symptoms. The theory behind this kind of preventative prescribing is that cats with FIV have impaired immune systems and therefore need antibiotics to protect them from secondary infections.
This strategy is flawed, and it does NOT work.

Antibiotics are designed to treat bacterial infections. They have no effect on fungal or viral infections. FIV is a viral infection, so antibiotics do not slow its progression in any way. Furthermore, when antibiotics are used for extended periods, they can actually weaken the immune system and leave FIV+ cats more prone to secondary infections.

The intestines contain healthy bacteria that are essential for digestion, proper nutrient absorption, and keeping harmful bacteria in check. Antibiotics, even when properly used, can kill these essential bacteria. Once the good bacteria have been damaged or destroyed, the door is open for harmful, potentially infectious bacteria in the intestines to flourish.

Through my work with FIV+ cats, I have learned that antibiotics become less effective when used repeatedly. With each course, bacteria grow resistant to antibiotics, the cat's immune system is further impaired, and infections become harder to treat. In the end, you are left with an ailing cat who has an infection that doesn't respond to antibiotics.

Four months before Jac was diagnosed with FIV, he began suffering from repeated sinus infections. Our local medical vet prescribed antibiotics, and the first two infections responded quite well. After that, it became increasingly difficult for Jac to recover, and the antibiotics no longer had any effect. Jac's upper respiratory infections were growing steadily worse, he was in danger of developing pneumonia, and medical vets we consulted had no means of treating him. If we hadn't been able to find a holistic practitioner who could treat Jac's infection, he most likely would have died.

This is another advantage of holistic treatments over antibiotics. Unlike antibiotics that become less and less effective with each course, natural treatments do not generally diminish in their effectiveness with repeated use. As a result, natural treatments are often more effective than antibiotics in helping immune-deficient cats conquer recurrent infections.

GUIDELINES FOR SAFE ANTIBIOTIC USE

When caring for FIV+ cats, it is essential to use antibiotics very carefully. There are some simple guidelines you can follow to help assure that your cat does not receive excessive or inappropriate antibiotics.

- If possible, work with a skilled vet who has medical and holistic training. These specialists can determine if your cat truly needs an antibiotic.

- Any time your cat is placed on an antibiotic, begin administering acidophilus supplements immediately. These products can help to restore the normal balance of bacteria in the intestines, and also address the diarrhea and profusely foul smelling gas or stools that often result from antibiotic treatment.

- Watch for side effects. Antibiotics can cause stomach upset and vomiting. If your cat develops these symptoms, it may be necessary for your vet to select a different antibiotic.

- Complete the entire course of the antibiotic. Many pet owners stop antibiotic therapies early because their cats seem to look and feel better. Stopping an antibiotic early can leave behind resistant bacteria that will cause future infections. The only time you should stop an antibiotic early is when the animal is experiencing side effects and doesn't appear to be tolerating the drug. If this occurs, you should contact your vet immediately and discuss other treatment options.

- Look for signs of improvement. If your cat does not get better while receiving antibiotics, there are a few important possibilities you should explore.

    - Re-examine the diagnosis: Your cat may not be suffering from a bacterial infection. Fungal and viral infections do not respond to antibiotic treatment.

    - Make sure you have the right antibiotic: No antibiotic is right for every infection. If your cat is not getting better, your vet may wish to try a different antibiotic.

    - Look for underlying problems: Work with your vet to determine if your cat's infections are being caused by an underlying problem. Allergies, for example, can cause bacterial skin infections that will reoccur until the problem is correctly diagnosed and treated.

- Some cats cannot tolerate antibiotics at all. For these animals, alternative forms of treatment are required.

STEROIDS

Steroids are among the most frequently misused medications in the field of veterinary medicine. Veterinarians use these powerful drugs because they can provide fast, short-term relief of itching, inflammation, swelling, and pain (specifically pain caused by swelling).

Unfortunately, steroids have potentially serious consequences, and they do nothing to address the root causes of illness. They merely suppress symptoms for a period of time. Even worse, steroids can actually drive an illness deeper into an animal's system, leading to additional medical problems.

Another drawback is that doctors frequently prescribe steroids without first making a correct diagnosis. The end result is that many pets receive incorrect or improper treatment for months or years before their medical condition is correctly identified and treated. When given to an FIV+ cat, steroids can have uniquely devastating effects.

Steroids work by suppressing the immune system, the last thing a cat with FIV can afford. In fact, steroids can suppress an FIV+ cat's immune system to the point where the animal simply can't recover. Many pet owners and holistic practitioners have come to me with heartbreaking stories of FIV+ cats who could have been saved through natural treatments if only their immune systems hadn't been irreparably damaged by steroids.

Despite the risks, many doctors still prescribe steroids for cats with FIV. This is endemic of what is taking place in the medical community at this time. Steroids have come to be regarded as miracle drugs, and there is a growing tendency among many medical professionals to prescribe these medications for any disease or symptom. Countless FIV+ cats have lost their lives as a result of inappropriate steroid use.

Whenever I am caring for a cat with FIV, I always start by looking for natural treatments that don't have the immunosuppressive effects of steroids. I have found that in most cases, dietary improvements, vitamin therapies, homeopathy, and natural immune stimulants can provide safe, effective results.

INTERFERON

Interferon is an anti-viral drug routinely prescribed by medical vets as a treatment for FIV. The goal of interferon therapy is to reduce the level of viral agents in the infected cat's body, thus allowing the animal's immune system to fend off the disease.

Cats, like humans, produce interferon naturally. It is a normal part of the immune response to viral infections. The interferon prescribed by veterinarians is a synthetic copy of the substance the body manufactures naturally.

When prescribing interferon, veterinarians often tell pet owners it is completely harmless – no more dangerous than a cat treat. The reasoning behind this is that cats produce interferon naturally, and therefore, it should be universally safe. Unfortunately, this simply isn't true.

The amount of interferon naturally produced in the body is quite small. When veterinarians attempt to artificially supplement a cat's interferon production, the amount of interferon in the animal's body is significantly increased, and side effects can result.

Some cats experience stiffness, aching muscles, severe fatigue, vomiting, and other flu-like symptoms from interferon. I have corresponded with many pet owners whose FIV+ cats got dramatically worse after being placed on this drug. Medical and holistic vets I have consulted reported some similar experiences. The bottom line is that there are potential side effects to interferon therapy.

I would be doing a disservice if I didn't point out that some FIV+ cats have benefited from interferon therapy. There are pet owners who credit interferon with saving their cats from FIV. For these animals, interferon therapy has obviously been quite beneficial.

Other cats receive no benefits from interferon. The drug doesn’t harm them, but it doesn’t help them either.

By medical standards, the use of interferon in cats is a relatively new practice. There is still a great deal to be learned about its effects. This may explain why the medical community cannot account for the widely varying results from interferon therapy in cats.

I cannot tell you if you should or should not pursue interferon therapy for your cat. Personally, I don't use interferon in my work with FIV+ cats because I'm simply not comfortable with it. Furthermore, natural treatments offer an abundance of options for combating viruses, supporting the immune system, and keeping FIV+ cats healthy. I would never even consider interferon before exhausting these safe, effective methods first.

OTHER SERIOUS FELINE DISEASES: Feline Leukemia (FeLV) and Feline Infectious Peritonitis (FIP)

Feline Leukemia (FeLV) and Feline Infectious Peritonitis (FIP) are two serious diseases that pet owners often confuse with FIV. All three are viral diseases that attack the immune system, and they have similar names. However, they are completely different diseases.

FIV is by far the least contagious of these diseases and is also the most treatable. Unfortunately, I've heard from pet owners who euthanized their FIV+ cats, mistakenly believing them to be infected with a deadly, highly contagious disease. My hope is that the following information will resolve any confusion and illustrate the differences between these diseases and FIV.

<u>Feline Leukemia (FeLV)</u>: This disease is a leading cause of death among cats. It invades the cells of the immune system and reduces production of white blood cells. These vital cells serve as the control center of the immune system. With the presence of the feline leukemia virus, the white cells become "confused" and can no longer efficiently fight infection. Some cats with feline leukemia also develop tumors and an aggressive form of cancer called "lymphosarcoma" that attacks the lymph-system.

FeLV is spread through saliva, mucus, urine, feces, and blood. Some vets recommend that FeLV+ cats live alone or with other cats who also carry the disease. There are pet owners who have successfully maintained multiple cat households without incident, but the risk of transmission does exist in such living environments.[3]

Holistic practitioners have enjoyed varying degrees of success in treating cats afflicted with feline leukemia. Nonetheless, the disease kills many cats each year.

Feline Infectious Peritonitis (FIP): This vicious disease is highly contagious and can be spread through saliva and feces, sharing of bedding, food and water bowls or litter pans. The disease is rare in the general cat population, but occurs in higher numbers in cat shelters and catteries. Those most at risk are cats under the age of two, over the age of ten, and those fighting infection or other illness.

There are two common forms of FIP: wet and dry. Wet form FIP is uniquely devastating. Blood vessels throughout the body leak fluids, which accumulate in the chest or abdomen. This causes pain, as well as difficulty breathing. Once the disease reaches this stage, it is most often fatal.

Dry FIP may develop more slowly, but it is serious. Although fluid build-up is minimal, there is weight loss, fever and anemia. Other symptoms may include kidney and liver failure, vomiting, diarrhea, and a variety of neurological symptoms ranging from balance problems to paralysis and seizures.[4]

There is no reliable test for FIP. Any cat that has been exposed to the disease will have antibodies that can trigger a false-positive test result.

Many holistic vets have found that despite their best efforts, chances of surviving FIP are no better than fifty percent. The medical and holistic communities are working to find viable treatments for this deadly disease.

COMMON PROBLEMS

FIV can affect cats in many ways. For this reason, it simply isn't possible to write a book that discusses every conceivable symptom the disease can produce. Instead, I have attempted to cover the problems I encounter most frequently.

I have received dozens and, in some cases, hundreds of emails about each of the following problems:

- eye problems
- ear problems
- nasal congestion
- mouth problems
- kidney disease
- liver disease
- constipation
- diarrhea
- vomiting
- advanced FIV

This information is not intended to replace professional medical guidance. No book can do that. My goal is to direct pet owners to the best possible information and avoid common pitfalls.

EYE PROBLEMS

When their immune systems are compromised, FIV+ cats often develop eye problems. Although these are common FIV symptoms, I always urge pet owners to exercise caution.

The eyes are delicate, and serious damage can occur quickly. Redness, swelling, or irritation can indicate hemorrhaging, a severe infection, or a foreign body in the eye. If such a problem goes undetected, your cat could lose the use of the affected eye.

Visiting your local vet for a thorough examination of your cat's eyes is always a wise precaution. Once the possibility of a serious eye problem has been ruled out, it is safe to proceed with other treatment options.

I regularly see FIV+ cats with eye drainage, and in some cases, a gland resembling a third eyelid covers a portion of one or both eyes. The discomfort of these symptoms often causes cats to squint. This condition is known as conjunctivitis, and it is usually the result of a herpes virus.

Medical vets often prescribe antibiotics for FIV+ cats with conjunctivitis. This approach is generally ineffective because antibiotics are not designed to kill viruses.

L-Lysine, the amino acid used for treating herpes outbreaks in humans, has proven effective in treating cats with herpes-related eye problems. Holistic practitioners often recommend oral L-Lysine doses of 250 milligrams twice per day. Many cats experience substantial improvements in less than a week while receiving this supplement.

Jac recovered from conjunctivitis on a regimen of dietary nutrition and vitamin supplements, including vitamins A, E, and C. Many other FIV+ cats I've cared for have enjoyed similar recoveries, but topical treatments are sometimes required to soothe badly irritated eyes. Saline eye drops such as artificial tears can help to moisten dry eyes and relieve minor irritation. For more advanced conditions, prescription eye products are occasionally needed.

Oral steroids pose many risks to FIV+ cats and should be avoided. However, short courses of steroidal eye drops or creams can be useful, especially when fast relief of swelling and irritation is needed to prevent permanent damage. Unlike oral steroids, these topical products are not absorbed into the bloodstream and subsequently pose no threat to the immune system.

I have used steroid-based eye products to treat a number of FIV+ cats with advanced eye problems. Several months ago, a local family asked me to help with a newly adopted FIV+ cat named George.

As a homeless cat, George went untreated, and his conjunctivitis reached a critical stage. Both eyes were irritated. A swollen, bloody red gland covered the bottom half of his left eye. The local vet determined that George was in danger of losing his eye if the swelling couldn't be reduced quickly.

Steroid-based eye creams were prescribed, and George began to improve over the next few days. Less than two weeks later, George's eye was looking quite healthy.

Topical steroids are not a cure for conjunctivitis. They merely provide temporary relief of symptoms, and long-term use can damage the eyes. To prevent George from experiencing a reoccurrence of conjunctivitis, and to keep his FIV in check, I placed him on a regimen of vitamins and

L-Lysine. I also made improvements to his diet. This regimen should be provided to any FIV+ cat with eye problems, whether steroids are used or not.

EAR PROBLEMS

Feline ear canals provide an ideal breeding ground for yeast and bacterial infections. Medical vets often treat ear infections by thoroughly cleaning the infected cat's ears and administering steroid-based or antibiotic eardrops to kill the infection and reduce any localized inflammation. This form of treatment works well for many ear infections.

FIV+ cats, because of their impaired immune systems, are susceptible to recurrent ear infections. Boosting the immune system often resolves these problems, but some cats require ongoing treatment.

Parasites, usually mites, can also irritate the ears. Unlike fleas, mites are too small to see without a microscope. Only a veterinarian can diagnose mites. The problem can often be resolved with a thorough cleaning of the infested cat's ears. Don't attempt this procedure yourself, as you could easily rupture your cat's eardrums.

Once your cat's ears are cleaned, you'll probably need to follow up with several days of eardrops. It's usually best to let a trained professional recommend products for continued treatment, but I would urge caution. Some veterinarians use powerful injectable medications that can have harmful side effects. One of my own cats nearly died when the vet gave him a shot of a potent anti-parasitic drug intended to kill mites.

Holistic practitioners often treat mites with natural products. Neem oil from Ayush Herbs (800.925.1371) and Ark Naturals Ears All Right (888.937.6677) are two excellent choices. Use as directed.

Foreign objects occasionally cause ear problems. Plant parts and other debris become lodged in the ear, resulting in irritation. In such cases, the irritation typically won't subside until the offending object is removed.

Ear problems are sometimes the result of a systemic illness. In such cases, topical treatments like eardrops generally aren't effective. At best, such products offer short-term symptom relief. Addressing the root cause of your cat's ear problems is the only way to achieve long-term relief.

Food allergies are a common cause of feline ear problems. Cats with allergies often experience a sudden reddening or flushing of their ears immediately after eating. In some cases, these animals also shake their heads and rub their ears against furniture or the floor in an attempt to relieve itching. NOTE: Liver disease and kidney disease can also produce these symptoms.

The assistance of a skilled vet with holistic experience is often required to resolve food allergies. However, you can do your cat a favor by making the transition from commercial pet foods to a higher quality, less processed diet.

No matter what is causing your cat's ear problems, seek medical attention. The mechanism of the inner ear governs balance. Untreated ear problems can cause severe dizziness and impaired coordination.

Furthermore, the severe itching and irritation caused by ear problems often compels cats to scratch their ears with their hind claws. I've actually seen cats scratch holes in their ears, including one animal who needed to have his ears surgically reattached. With prompt treatment and follow-up care, these problems can be avoided.

NASAL CONGESTION

Many cats with FIV suffer from chronic nasal congestion, usually as the result of upper respiratory and sinus infections. Because these infections tend to be viral in origin, antibiotics typically aren't helpful.

When given to cats with FIV, antibiotics often become less effective with repeated use. Even if your cat has a bacterial infection that initially responds to antibiotics, these drugs probably won't continue to work well in the long-term.

In the months before Jac was diagnosed with FIV, he developed reoccurring sinus infections accompanied by thick green drainage in both nostrils. Our local medical vet attempted to treat Jac with multiple courses of antibiotics. The first two infections responded well. After that, the antibiotics no longer had any effect, and Jac's sinus infections were growing steadily worse. At this point, our medical vet informed us he had no means of treating Jac. If we hadn't found a holistic practitioner with alternative treatment methods, Jac probably would have died.

What happened to Jac happens to many cats with FIV. Every week I receive emails from frightened pet owners with ailing FIV+ cats suffering from nasal congestion and upper respiratory infections that will no longer respond to antibiotics. Although antibiotics can be helpful for treating isolated infections that don't respond to natural treatments, these drugs generally aren't a good choice for treating FIV+ cats with reoccurring infections.

In addition to antibiotics, some medical veterinarians also attempt to treat nasal congestion with non-prescription drugs designed for humans, usually Benadryl or Sudafed. This is a mistake, and it can be dangerous.

Many over-the-counter preparations contain preservatives, artificial colors, and ingredients like sodium benzoate that are toxic to cats. They also contain flavorings that are strong enough to make some cats choke or foam at the mouth. There are other risks to these products as well.

Benadryl is an antihistamine commonly used to relieve human allergy symptoms. While the drug works well for this purpose, it is not appropriate for treating cats with nasal congestion. Benadryl has a dehydrating effect that can actually make nasal congestion worse. It dries up and thickens mucous in the sinuses, making it almost impossible to expel.

Another drawback is that Benadryl can cause significant increases in blood pressure and heart rate. In fact, cardiologists treating humans generally recommend against the use of Benadryl by patients with a history of heart attack or stroke. These same risks apply to cats.

Sudafed is not a good choice for cats either. It is an excellent decongestant, but it carries the same cardiac risks as Benadryl. In humans, Sudafed can cause substantial, potentially risky increases in blood pressure and heart rate. When it is given to a tiny animal like a cat, these risks are amplified considerably.

If your cat is struggling with persistent nasal congestion, it is important to address the root cause of the problem rather than just attempting to mask the symptoms. Remember, nasal congestion is most often the result of an infection, and it can also be an indication that your cat's immune system is faltering. Antibiotics and over-the-counter drugs will do nothing to bolster your cat's immune system, and any symptom relief they provide will be temporary at best.

There are safe, effective natural treatments available, but I have yet to find any single product or approach that consistently relieves nasal congestion. In most cases, combinations of natural therapies are required.

Anytime I am confronted with FIV+ cats suffering from nasal congestion, I start by examining their diet and looking for ways to increase their nutritional intake. This may sound like common sense, but pet owners and veterinarians frequently overlook dietary nutrition while caring for FIV+ cats.

On a regular basis, I receive letters from pet owners who are feeding their cats a diet comprised entirely of grocery store or vet clinic cat food, and they don't understand why the animals aren't getting well. FIV+ cats have the best chance to recover from upper respiratory infections with quality food-source nutrition.

As I learned while caring for Jac, feeding an FIV+ cat who has a stuffy nose can be difficult. When cats can't smell, they typically won't eat. During Jac's worst upper respiratory infections, there were times when he would only eat highly aromatic foods such as cod, tuna, or roasted delicatessen chicken, because these were the only foods he could smell. I've served these same foods to many other ailing FIV+ cats I've cared for with very good results.

While the importance of proper nutrition cannot be overstated, additional tools are required to resolve most cases of nasal congestion. Vitamin C, for example, has proven invaluable to immune-compromised cats with upper respiratory difficulties. Holistic practitioners commonly use this supplement to treat FIV+ cats for colds, sinus infections, and a variety of other illnesses. Without exception, I give vitamin C to every FIV+ cat under my care.

When given in large enough doses, vitamin C stimulates the immune system, reduces swelling (including swelling of the nasal passages), and acts as an antihistamine.[5] Holistic veterinarians regularly treat cats with doses of 200 to 250 milligrams per day or more. If you decide to use this approach, you should start with smaller doses. Increasing the dose of vitamin C gradually will reduce the chance of stomach upset. You will also have to determine your cat's bowel tolerance (the point where loose stools and gas occur and you must reduce the dose of vitamin C).

Health food stores across the country offer many forms of vitamin C. One excellent product is Mega C from Orthomolecular Specialties (www.belfield.com). Mega C is a high quality vitamin C supplement that also contains a blend of vitamins and minerals, including vitamins A and E. This is important because vitamin C is most effective when used in combination with vitamins A and E.

Like vitamin C, vitamins A and E help to support the immune system. Vitamin A is especially useful for cats with nasal congestion because it helps to maintain healthy mucous membranes.

Upper respiratory infections are often the product of a herpes virus, and the amino acid L-Lysine can be helpful. A growing number of holistic practitioners are using L-Lysine to treat FIV+ cats for upper respiratory infections. Doses of 250 milligrams twice daily are safe and well tolerated by most cats.

In addition to vitamins and supplements, homeopathic remedies can be highly effective in treating cats suffering from nasal congestion. FIV+ cats with sinus infections often recover after receiving homeopathic remedies. There are many good remedies, but one in particular is recommended by holistic practitioners I have consulted.

The homeopathic remedy Infection is available through http://pets4homeopathy.com and www.newtonlabs.net . This product is a combination or “shotgun” remedy designed to help fight a variety of bacterial and viral infections. For stubborn nasal congestion, some practitioners also recommend Nose Relief – a combination homeopathic remedy from Homeopet (www.homeopet.com).

Animals Apawthecary (animalessentials.com) offers Eye & Nose Drops to help dilute nasal mucous, fight infection, and soothe swollen nasal tissues. They also make OL-Immune and Echinacea/Goldenseal Blend – potent herbals that can be used for tough infections that don’t respond to homeopathy.

Dehydration can be another factor in nasal congestion. Healthy cats tend to be very poor water drinkers. Cats who are sick generally drink even less.

Drinking fluids helps to hydrate the tissues of the sinuses and dilute mucous secretions. When an animal drinks only minimal fluids or stops drinking altogether, this can allow nasal mucous to become very thick and difficult to pass. In many cases, getting fluids into a cat (orally or through an IV) can help to ease nasal congestion.

The products and approaches I have described in this section work very well for many FIV+ cats. However, if you have taken all of the above-mentioned steps and haven’t seen an improvement in your cat’s condition, you most likely require the help of an experienced professional, preferably someone with medical as well as holistic experience.

MOUTH PROBLEMS

FIV+ cats often develop painful mouth problems. When the immune system is compromised, opportunistic bacteria and viruses in the mouth can flourish, resulting in inflamed gums, mouth sores, and tartar. Conventional treatments are generally ineffective.

One common medical strategy involves surgically removing the infected cat's teeth and administering large doses of antibiotics, steroids, and interferon. I have yet to hear from even one pet owner who saw an improvement in his or her FIV+ cat through this approach. More often than not, this treatment strategy fails to resolve mouth problems, and it leaves the infected animal's immune system even more depleted.

To the best of my knowledge, there is no quick fix for mouth problems. There are, however, treatment options that have proven helpful to many FIV+ cats.

L-Lysine is essential for any cat with mouth problems. This amino acid has proven effective in treating humans for herpes outbreaks and mouth sores. In fact, it often works better than prescription drugs intended for this purpose.

Many FIV+ cats experience dramatic recoveries from mouth problems while being treated with L-Lysine. I prefer to use the L-Lysine supplements that are available in capsule form at most natural supplement stores. The capsules pull apart easily, and you can sprinkle the L-Lysine powder into some baby food or finely diced wet cat food.

You can also mix L-Lysine powder with some liquid and squirt it down your cat's throat in the same manner you would administer a prescription medication. This option works well for cats who are experiencing too much mouth pain to handle solid food.

L-Lysine is safe and well tolerated by most cats. When treating FIV+ cats for mouth problems, holistic practitioners often use doses of 250 milligrams twice daily. All of Jac's doctors supported this approach.

In addition to L-Lysine, vitamin C can help to maintain healthy teeth and gums. Studies by holistic practitioners have shown that cats receiving supplemental vitamin C have fewer mouth problems and healthier teeth. Doses of 200 to 250 milligrams per day or more are commonly used.

Cats with mouth problems respond best when vitamin C is used in combination with vitamins A and E. Vitamin A helps to maintain healthy skin throughout the body, including the gums. Vitamin E is known for helping to rejuvenate the immune system. Jac and many other FIV+ cats I've cared for responded well to this combination of vitamins.

Pycnogenol and CoQ10 have proven highly beneficial to many FIV+ cats suffering from mouth sores and inflamed gums. These powerful supplements can reduce swelling and stimulate the immune system.

When administering pycnogenol, doses of 10 milligrams per day are often used, but some practitioners recommend 1 milligram per pound of body weight. CoQ10 can cause stomach upset, and some practitioners recommend two small daily doses of 10 milligrams each. Pycnogenol and CoQ10 may be administered in the same fashion as L-Lysine – mixed in moist food, or squirted down the throat in a liquid solution. NOTE: Pycnogenol and CoQ10 are most effective when used in conjunction with vitamins A, E, and C.

B-complex vitamins can help to fight gingivitis and maintain healthy gums. However, veterinarians caring for cats with mouth problems often overlook these important vitamins. The B-complex supplements made for humans are not suitable for cats. These products are extremely bitter, and they can make cats choke, foam at the mouth, or vomit. Orthomolecular Specialties (www.belfield.com) has developed a B-complex supplement for cats. Many companies offer such products, but this is the one I am most familiar with.

To provide comfort and stimulate healing of sore gums, I highly recommend Vital Liquid, also sold by Orthomolecular Specialties. This product is especially effective when applied directly to irritated gums and administered internally.

Vital Liquid works well for many cats, but additional treatments are sometimes required. Holistic practitioners often recommend Echinacea-Goldenseal tinctures, applied directly to the affected area twice daily with a Q-tip or sterile gauze. Herb Pharm (http://www.herb-pharm.com/) makes an alcohol-free, glycerin-based tincture that many cats tolerate. Animals Apawthecary (www.animalessentials.com) makes a product called FidoDent that can also be used in this fashion.

Besides providing your cat with a nutritionally rich diet, it is also important to make sure that he or she is actually eating. FIV+ cats with mouth problems sometimes reach a point where they are no longer able to chew their food.

I have received several heart-wrenching emails from pet owners whose FIV+ cats literally starved to death in front of their food dishes. To avoid this tragedy, I always made sure that Jac had access to a wide variety of soft, moist foods at each meal. This assured there was always something on Jac's plate that he was physically capable of eating. Cats with mouth problems frequently stop drinking because the sensation of water touching their teeth and gums is simply too painful. If your cat has been plagued with mouth problems for an extended period, he or she may be dehydrated and require a saline IV.

In addition to supplements and dietary nutrition, oral rinses are sometimes necessary. Immune-compromised cats often develop an excessive buildup of germs and bacteria on their teeth and gums. Oral rinses can help to cleanse the mouth and jumpstart the healing process. I have cared for a few FIV+ cats who were unable to recover until their mouths and teeth were thoroughly cleaned in a veterinary setting.

There are also occasions when individual teeth need to be pulled. When severe damage or decay exposes the root nerves of a tooth, the animal may experience substantial pain until it is removed. Just remember that summarily pulling all of your cat's teeth will not solve his or her FIV-related mouth problems.

Mouth problems are systemic in origin and must be addressed as such. Supporting the immune system and fighting infection through dietary nutrition, proper supplementation, and oral hygiene are the most effective ways to contain or resolve mouth problems.

KIDNEY DISEASE

I have encountered many FIV+ cats afflicted with kidney disease, a leading cause of death among cats.

The kidneys filter wastes from the blood, allowing them to be excreted from the body during urination. When disease impairs these vital organs, they lose their ability to filter the blood, and internal poisoning can result.

The poor quality of commercial cat foods has been directly linked to steady increases in feline kidney disease. These foods contain inferior sources of protein and chemical additives that the kidneys labor to process.

Feeding your cat nothing but dry food can be dangerous. Jac's doctors explained that cats in the wild survive by eating mice, birds, and other prey whose bodies have a substantial fluid content. Dry cat food simply doesn't offer the moisture content necessary to maintain healthy kidneys. This is why so many young cats are developing kidney damage previously seen only in the most elderly cats.

Cats in the early stages of kidney disease often improve when they are switched from dry cat food diets to canned or homemade food and raw meat. The increased moisture and rich nutritional content of these foods is often enough to promote improved kidney function. In fact, such diets can prevent many cases of kidney disease.

Medical vets often recommend low-protein diets for cats. Their rationale is that high-protein diets cause kidney disease. Recent studies suggest this isn't the case. Commercial pet foods contain indigestible proteins that are extremely hard on the kidneys. Quality sources of protein, however, can be beneficial.

Another medical strategy for treating feline kidney disease involves steroids. These drugs are often prescribed to prevent swelling, reduce pain, and stimulate appetite. This approach can be problematic, especially when applied to an FIV+ cat.

Steroids do nothing to repair the kidneys, and they can cause damage in the long term. Furthermore, steroids suppress the immune system. These drugs can leave an immune-compromised animal vulnerable to infection and disease.

Dr. Robert Goldstein, VMD, has developed a comprehensive, user-friendly approach that includes dietary guidelines, supplements, and homeopathic remedies.

Dr. Goldstein's potentially life-saving treatment strategy is available to pet owners in "The Veterinarians' Guide To Natural Remedies for Cats" by Martin Zucker (pages 198-199), © 1999. Additional information about Dr. Goldstein's services may be obtained at http://healingcenterforanimals.com/ .

Tanya's Feline Chronic Renal Failure Information Centre, http://www.felinecrf.org/ , is packed with information about medical and holistic treatments for kidney disease. There are also two Yahoo groups with diverse memberships that can offer support and suggestions.

http://health.groups.yahoo.com/group/Pets4Homeopathy/

http://groups.yahoo.com/group/Feline-CRF-Support/

LIVER DISEASE

The liver performs many essential functions. It helps the body efficiently make use of fats, proteins, and carbohydrates, and also removes toxins from the blood and sends them to the kidneys to be processed.

Liver disease can have serious consequences, and prompt treatment is recommended. Unfortunately, liver disease is often misdiagnosed. Some cats suffer vomiting and other symptoms for weeks before the condition is correctly diagnosed.

A woman from Texas recently contacted me about her FIV+ cat who was throwing up several times per week. Over a period of four months, this woman spent hundreds of dollars having her cat re-hydrated and treated with prescription drugs to suppress vomiting. I referred her to a skilled vet with medical and holistic experience. Her cat was immediately diagnosed with liver disease, and once the condition was properly treated, the vomiting stopped.

Medical vets often attempt to treat liver disease with steroids, which can be dangerous for cats with FIV. Many holistic vets use a combination of two natural treatments for cats with liver disease. The first of these approaches involves homeopathy.

Liver Detox, available at http://pets4homeopathy.com/, is a combination homeopathic remedy designed to help detoxify the liver and restore normal function. This product is safe and works well for many cats. King Bio (www.kingbio.com) also makes a Liver Detox remedy.

In addition to homeopathic remedies, the herbal supplement milk thistle has shown a remarkable ability to heal and regenerate the liver. It is generally regarded as essential for any cat experiencing liver problems.

There are many forms of milk thistle available in capsule form at health food stores. I prefer these because the capsules pull apart and the contents can be sprinkled into a flavorful moist food.

The natural treatments I've described work well for many cats. Nevertheless, it is always wise to seek professional guidance when caring for an FIV+ cat afflicted with liver disease.

CONSTIPATION

Some cats, like humans, chronically experience constipation. Hairballs and dietary problems are two of the most common causes. Elderly cats are especially prone to constipation because their colons lack the strength to properly move stool. Fortunately, most cases of constipation can be prevented or treated without using harsh prescription drugs.

Vetbasis Hairball Gel is one of many good products available at pet stores. It helps to prevent hairballs and also lubricates the colon, allowing stools to slide through more easily. Administering this product once per week is often enough to keep hairballs in check and prevent constipation.

Holistic practitioners sometimes use vitamin C to relieve constipation and keep cats regular. You may recall that large doses of vitamin C often cause loose runny stools.

Jac had very few problems with constipation because the vitamins in his sports drink kept his stools soft enough to pass with minimal effort. None of the FIV+ cats under my care have ever developed constipation while receiving the sports drink.

Dietary changes can also be helpful. If you feed your cat only dry food, that could be causing the animal's constipation. These foods are dehydrating, and they often contain ingredients that are binding.

Canned or homemade cat foods and real meat provide dietary moisture that can make stools easier to expel. Jac, like all of my cats, received a diet of dry food, wet food, and real meat. I believe this is another reason he had so few problems staying regular.

Some practitioners recommend a small amount of dietary bran or oatmeal for cats who are predisposed to chronic constipation. I am reluctant to advocate this approach because excessive dietary fiber can be binding, especially when given to a cat who is already constipated. Adding additional roughage to your cat's diet can be helpful, but it must be done carefully.

Phytomucil, made by Animals Apawthecary (www.animalessentials.com), contains slippery elm and other carefully selected herbs that help to relieve constipation without side effects. Many practitioners recommend this product, which can also be used to treat diarrhea.

I have spoken to holistic vets who recommend a product called Capra Mineral Whey, available from Christine's Cleanse Corner (877.673.0224). This whole food supplement, made from goat's milk, works well for treating constipation.

Unlike harsh prescription drugs, Capra Mineral Whey is safe for long-term use and poses no threat to the immune system. It also contains an abundance of minerals and helps to soothe the intestines.

I have seen a few cats with advanced constipation that required medical intervention. Two of these cases are noteworthy.

Tiger was an FIV+ cat from Michigan. He was ill for several days and became badly dehydrated. Due to his minimal fluid intake, the fecal matter is his colon became dry, firm, and impassable.

To restore Tiger's normal bowel function, a local vet administered prescription grade laxatives, a saline IV, and a series of enemas.

Another cat, Corey, belonged to a local family. He was very sick, and his symptoms were not consistent with FIV. While I was holding Corey, he vomited a large quantity of fecal matter, and we rushed him to a nearby vet clinic.

As it turned out, Corey had a bowel obstruction preventing any stool from being passed. His bowels backlogged until he was literally vomiting feces. Surgery was performed to remove the obstruction, and Corey remained hospitalized for more than a week as doctors struggled to detoxify his system.

I am happy to report that Corey and Tiger made full recoveries. However, they both could have died if their owners had waited any longer to seek medical care. If your cat has an ongoing problem, don't hesitate to seek medical attention. Constipation, left untreated, can become serious.

DIARRHEA

I often receive email about FIV+ cats with diarrhea. This can be a challenging problem to deal with because there are many possible causes.

Diarrhea, like vomiting, can be brought on when cats eat something they shouldn't. One of my own cats, Felix, developed diarrhea after dining on a rotten animal carcass he found under a bush in our backyard.

Commercial pet foods are another common cause. The chemical additives and poor sources of meat in these foods can upset the gastrointestinal system, resulting in diarrhea. Parasites, as well as viral and bacterial infections, can also have this effect.

Pet owners often contact me after their cats have received multiple courses of antibiotics. These drugs can disrupt the balance of healthy bacteria in the colon, resulting in foul smelling gas, and in some cases, diarrhea.

Jac's doctors recommended fasting for cats with acute diarrhea because eating can further irritate the digestive tract and make the problem worse. Many holistic practitioners advocate this approach, allowing water but no food for a period of twenty-four hours. At the end of the fast, offer a small amount of bland food before resuming regular meals.

In addition to fasting, every holistic practitioner I've dealt with has recommended probiotics for cats with diarrhea. Supplements like acidophilus help to restore the normal balance of healthy intestinal bacteria, which is often enough to resolve the problem and prevent future flare-ups.

Used in combination with probiotics, homeopathic remedies can be helpful. Nux Vomica, a single homeopathic remedy, can calm the gastrointestinal tract and curb episodes of diarrhea (see page 69). There are also many combination remedies available. Diarrhea & Gas, available through http://pets4homeopathy.com/ and www.newtonlabs.net, is the product I'm most familiar with.

During bouts of diarrhea, supplements like vitamin C should be withheld because they can further loosen stools and make the problem worse. Other supplements, however, can be helpful.

Slippery elm is an herb often used by holistic practitioners to relive diarrhea. It has a high mucilage content, allowing it to coat and soothe inflamed mucous membranes in the bowel and give body to otherwise loose runny stools.

Ongoing diarrhea can deplete a cat and cause severe rectal irritation. It can also be an indication of a more serious medical condition like liver disease, kidney disease, or irritable bowel syndrome. Anytime diarrhea fails to resolve itself within a day, seeking professional help is wise.

NOTE: If diarrhea is violent, repeated, or accompanied by vomiting, DO NOT wait. Withhold all food and contact your veterinarian immediately.

VOMITING

In many cases, vomiting starts when cats eat something they shouldn't. Cats are famous for nibbling on houseplants, chunks of spoiled meat from trashcans, and other items that can trigger episodes of vomiting.

Fasting is important if your cat has thrown up more than once in the same day. When cats throw up, their instincts often drive them to replace the lost food and fluids by eating and drinking. This usually leads to more vomiting.

When cats vomit more than a few times, they are often unable to stop – which can lead to dehydration. I have found that once an animal reaches this point, IV fluids and medication are often required to break the cycle. This happened to my youngest cat, Felix.

My father placed some old cat food in our driveway for the crows to eat. Felix found this spoiled food and ate a generous portion. Within hours, he started throwing up. While I was on the phone asking our vet for advice, Felix ran to the food dish and gorged. Moments later, he was vomiting again, seemingly unable to stop. My family and I rushed Felix to the hospital where he received IV fluids and prescription drugs to stop his vomiting.

What happened to Felix can often be avoided by withholding food and water for a period of twenty-four hours. This allows an agitated stomach time to settle. Homeopathic remedies can also aid this process. Nux Vomica 30C, available at most health food stores, relieves nausea and helps to calm an upset stomach. Some practitioners administer this remedy twice daily for three to four days — or more frequently if the episode is severe.

At the end of a fast, it is wise to start with small amounts of a very bland food that isn't likely to cause stomach upset. Baby food works well for this purpose.

Slippery elm, a nutrient-rich herb, can also be introduced at the conclusion of a fast to soothe the digestive tract and prevent additional episodes of vomiting. Most health food stores carry this herb in a powder form, which can be mixed with any moist food. Some practitioners recommend ¼ teaspoon twice per day.

Nux Vomica and slippery elm can be used together, and many holistic practitioners report excellent results when using this combination to treat cats who throw up regularly. However, there are times when these approaches simply aren't enough. Vomiting is sometimes caused by an underlying illness.

Commercial pet foods contain flavorings, preservatives, and poor quality meats that can wreak havoc on the digestive system. If your cat is allergic or sensitive to an ingredient in his or her food, vomiting will likely be recurrent until you change their diet.

Antibiotics are extremely hard on the stomach. Every month I receive email from pet owners whose cats have been throwing up since antibiotics were prescribed.

Liver disease is one of many serious medical conditions that can cause vomiting, and it is often misdiagnosed. I was recently contacted by a woman from Texas whose FIV+ cat had been throwing up several times per week. Over a period of four months, this woman spent hundreds of dollars having her cat re-hydrated and treated with prescription drugs to suppress vomiting. I referred her to a skilled vet with medical and holistic experience. Her cat was immediately diagnosed with liver disease, and once the condition was properly treated, the vomiting stopped.

Cats sometimes swallow foreign objects that can become lodged in the digestive tract and cause vomiting. While Felix was in the hospital, another cat was undergoing surgery to remove a Christmas decoration that he'd swallowed.

I always take vomiting seriously. The loss of fluids and nutrition that occurs during vomiting can be fatal in extreme cases. If your cat has an ongoing problem, don't hesitate to seek professional help.

NOTE: If vomiting is profuse, repeated, or accompanied by diarrhea, DO NOT wait. Withhold all food and contact your veterinarian immediately.

ADVANCED FIV: Protocols For Limp Dishrag Cats

One of the most frightening situations a pet owner faces is when a cat with advanced FIV suffers immune system failure and becomes overwhelmed by infection. This life-threatening stage can produce many symptoms, including severe fatigue. Pet owners often compare their lethargic FIV+ cats to limp dishrags. My cat, Jac, experienced this advanced form of FIV in July of 1995.

Jac's coat looked terrible, he'd lost weight and he had no appetite. He was running a fever, and he was uncharacteristically weak, spending his days lifelessly sprawled across his favorite sofa cushion. I felt helpless as I watched Jac's condition deteriorate, knowing he would die without effective treatment. I called dozens of medical vets, all of whom flatly stated that nothing could be done. Had I not persisted in seeking alternative treatment options, Jac would have died.

Advanced FIV, while sometimes fatal, does not have to mean an automatic death sentence. However, swift action and multiple techniques are required to save animals once the disease has progressed this far.

A routine medical examination is a good place to start. I've encountered FIV+ cats who were listless because of tumors, internal bleeding, cardiac difficulties, bowel obstructions, and other undiagnosed medical problems. Ruling out such possibilities before proceeding with treatment is wise.

Most cats with advanced FIV are at least marginally dehydrated and can benefit from a saline IV. Trying to re-hydrate these animals by squirting liquids down their throats doesn't always work. If your vet is willing to administer a saline IV, also request an injection of vitamin B-12 for your cat.

Holistic practitioners often use vitamin B-12 when treating FIV+ cats. This powerful vitamin can stimulate an ailing cat's immune system. Injections are preferred because vitamin B-12 is not absorbed well orally. During some of Jac's most critical illnesses, he received injections of vitamin B-12, and I am convinced he would not have recovered without it.

Ashwaganda, from Ayush Herbs (800.925.1371), can help to rejuvenate many ailing animals. I always use this potent herb when caring for so-called "limp dishrag" cats.

At this critical stage, homeopathic remedies are also required. Because multiple systems of the body are affected simultaneously, combination homeopathic remedies are recommended. A skilled holistic practitioner in New York has developed remedy protocols for cats with advanced FIV. The following remedies are available at http://pets4homeopathy.com and www.newtonlabs.net :

Pet Fatigue, Infection, Liver Detox, and *Bowel Discomfort.*

Administer two to three drops of each remedy, three times per day. Ideally, the remedies will be placed directly on the cat's tongue. After a few days, reduce to two times per day. Eventually decrease to once per day. Many cats experience a noticeable improvement within less than five days while receiving these remedies. By the end of a three-week period, the remedies can be terminated.

Providing your cat with nourishment is also essential. I've seen ailing FIV+ cats who would have been content to let themselves starve. If your cat won't eat voluntarily, force-feeding may be necessary.

Force-feeding is not meant to replace regular meals. The process is merely intended to help sustain the animal until he or she is well enough to resume eating. DO NOT attempt to forcibly administer massive quantities of food or fluids… your ailing cat might not be able to hold them down. Instead, give your cat small amounts of food twice per day.

I've had to force-feed several cats with advanced FIV. Chicken breast is easy to prepare and provides cats with valuable food-source nutrition. Canned chicken products, like those found in grocery store soup aisles, are NOT acceptable substitutes. These commercially prepared products are high in salt and often contain ingredients that are toxic to cats. Furthermore, they lack the nutritional content of fresh chicken.

To prepare chicken breast, thoroughly rinse the meat with cool water and place it in a glass baking dish. Add 2 ½ cups of water, and lightly salt the meat. Cover it with aluminum foil and bake at 425 degrees F for approximately one hour and twenty-five minutes. This process will cook the meat and create a rich yellow broth.

After it has cooled, pour the broth into a blender. Add generous slices of breast meat, making sure not to include any bone fragments. Blend until the meat is finely ground (the final product should be sufficiently liquefied to fit through a syringe).

Give your cat 3 cc's of this mixture two to three times per day. Remember not to squirt the broth down the middle of your cat's throat because it could get into the lungs. Always aim toward the back of the mouth and off to either side. If you have any questions, ask your veterinarian.

To avoid waste, freeze some of the broth for later use. Refrigerate the rest and discard the unused portion within forty-eight hours.

Vitamin supplements are also important. Nutri-Cal by Tomlyn (http://www.tomlyn.com/), is a high-calorie product that can help to sustain ailing cats and stimulate appetite.

Jac's sports drink has helped many cats. For cases of advanced FIV, I sometimes use a modified drink that is potent, but less likely to cause stomach upset.

The ingredients can be mixed in an ordinary baby food jar. Start with four tablespoons of milk and a heaping tablespoon of vanilla ice cream. For cats who don't tolerate milk, use one of the non-dairy milk substitutes sold in pet stores. Add 10,000 i.u. of vitamin A, 400 i.u of vitamin E, and 2,000 milligrams of vitamin C (Mega C works well for this purpose, but use whatever vitamin C product you have readily available). Shake thoroughly, until all of the ingredients are mixed.

Administer 3 cc's once per day. If your cat tolerates the drink, increase to twice per day. After three days, make a fresh batch. Once your cat is stronger, switch to Jac's regular sports drink.

These guidelines are not intended to replace professional care, nor do I offer any guarantees. In some cases, the disease progresses too far, permanent damage is done, and the animal can't be saved. However, Jac responded well to this form of treatment, and I've enjoyed favorable outcomes with many other FIV+ cats.

EUTHANASIA

When dealing with a serious disease like FIV, it is inevitable that euthanasia will be required for some cats. Major organ failures, neurological problems, breathing difficulties, and other painful ailments can arise unexpectedly. In such instances, when the animal's quality of life has been eroded and suffering will most likely be prolonged and without resolution, it is important to consider the compassionate choice of euthanasia.

I cannot emphasize strongly enough that euthanasia does not constitute a failure on the part of the pet owner... on the contrary. It takes tremendous strength and compassion to make this decision on behalf of your cat to spare him or her from ongoing and irreversible suffering. Knowing when to make this decision is not always easy.

Many medical doctors continue to prescribe euthanasia for any cat diagnosed with FIV, even when the animal is in good health and not showing symptoms. This is totally inappropriate and completely unnecessary. FIV, and most of the innumerable secondary illnesses it can produce, are generally treatable, and cats with this disease can live a high quality of life for an extended period. No cat should ever be put to sleep simply for testing FIV+.

Working with a highly skilled vet who has medical as well as holistic training can help you determine if your cat is truly terminal, or merely suffering from an illness for which the medical community does not yet have an answer. If you find yourself considering the possibility of euthanasia for your cat, I would urge you to seek out such a consultation. Otherwise, you could be left with painful, lingering doubts as to whether or not your cat would have recovered with another form of treatment.

I support the prolonging of life when there is a reasonable chance of recovery, and when the symptoms of illness can be well managed. When confronted with an ailing FIV+ cat, before I ever consider euthanasia, I will administer homeopathic remedies, nutritional therapies, and carefully selected medications with the hope of improving the animal's condition. As long as the animal's enjoyment of life outweighs the burden being imposed by his or her illness, I will continue to offer supportive care.

However, when an animal is enduring substantial pain and discomfort, and reasonable efforts cannot provide sufficient relief, I will consider euthanasia. Heart attacks, strokes, kidney failure and liver failure are some common problems that can abruptly put an animal on a path to a slow, painful, unavoidable death. When major systemic breakdowns like these occur, and quality of life has been lost, it is imperative to put your cat's needs ahead of your own by ending his or her suffering in the most humane and dignified manner possible.

GRIEF AND LOSS: The Death Of A Pet

No book about FIV would be complete without discussing grief and loss. FIV is a serious disease and some cats die, even with the best possible care.

You may need to make hard decisions about euthanasia. Once those decisions are made, your emotions may run a gamut – relief that your companion's suffering is over, guilt that you weren't able to do more, and feelings of loss and loneliness that can be difficult to bear.

It is impossible to predict how long you might feel this way. Those who don't understand may belittle your emotions by saying, "It was only a cat." This cold-hearted philosophy completely overlooks the important role pets play in our lives.

When we go through rough times (lost jobs, personal illness, poor relationships), our cats are there to provide unconditional love. In many respects, these gentle creatures compensate for our losses and become a vital lifeline. When that lifeline is severed, heart-wrenching grief can occur.

Grieving pet owners can benefit from sharing their feelings with someone who understands – a compassionate friend or a counselor. Also do something constructive in honor of your pet. Donate money or supplies to your local animal shelter (such facilities often have memorial programs). Hold a ceremony. Write a letter to your pet to include with burial or cremation. You need to do what's right for you, but be sure to do something. Formalizing your grief in this way will assure that your pet isn't forgotten. This process can also help you heal, but it will take time, so don't set unrealistic expectations for yourself.

The following links offer ceremony suggestions and a list of grief counselors who can provide understanding.

http://www.petloss.com/

http://www.imom.org/loss/

http://www.petloss.com/phones.htm

http://felinecrf.org/saying_goodbye.htm

http://www.aplb.org/

http://www.avma.org/careforanimals/animatedjourneys/goodbyefriend/plhotlines.asp

MY OWN EXPERIENCE: Jac's Death

Many pet owners have written, wanting to know how Jac died and what I did to cope. I hope this information will benefit others.

Jac died from age-related complications, not FIV. He was nearly eighteen years old when he suffered a massive heart attack and collapsed in our family dining room. His death was quick, and I was spared from euthanizing him, although I was prepared to do so.

I felt an obligation to bury Jac out of respect for the enormous role he played in my life for so many years. My father and I wrapped Jac in his favorite blanket and carried him to a sunny location in the backyard. Dad said a few words, and I took a lock of Jac's hair that I still keep on my bookshelf. Lowering Jac's lifeless body into the ground and covering him was an excruciating experience, but it helped me to accept that he was gone.

That evening, I lit a simple candle at Jac's gravesite. My parents' house felt empty. I left, only to find reminders of Jac seemingly everywhere. Grocery shopping was probably the activity I struggled with most. For months, every trip to the grocery store involved finding special meats and other delicacies for Jac. This duty was no longer required, and that took getting used to.

At first, I couldn't bear to visit Jac's grave, let alone decorate it. Then winter closed in. The ground froze hard like concrete, and snowstorms buried the yard. I knew the project would have to wait until spring.

Throughout the winter, I visited several garden stores, searching for flowers and statues that reflected Jac's personality. This was challenging because Jac was such a remarkable and complex individual.

During his youth, Jac was a rugged, street-brawling tomcat. Even in his final years, he occasionally chased large dogs from our yard and maintained his tough image. At the same time, Jac was loving and affectionate, possessing a charismatic personality that never went unnoticed by visitors to our home. He served as a loving father figure and mentor to our younger cats, while simultaneously fulfilling his role as a model family cat.

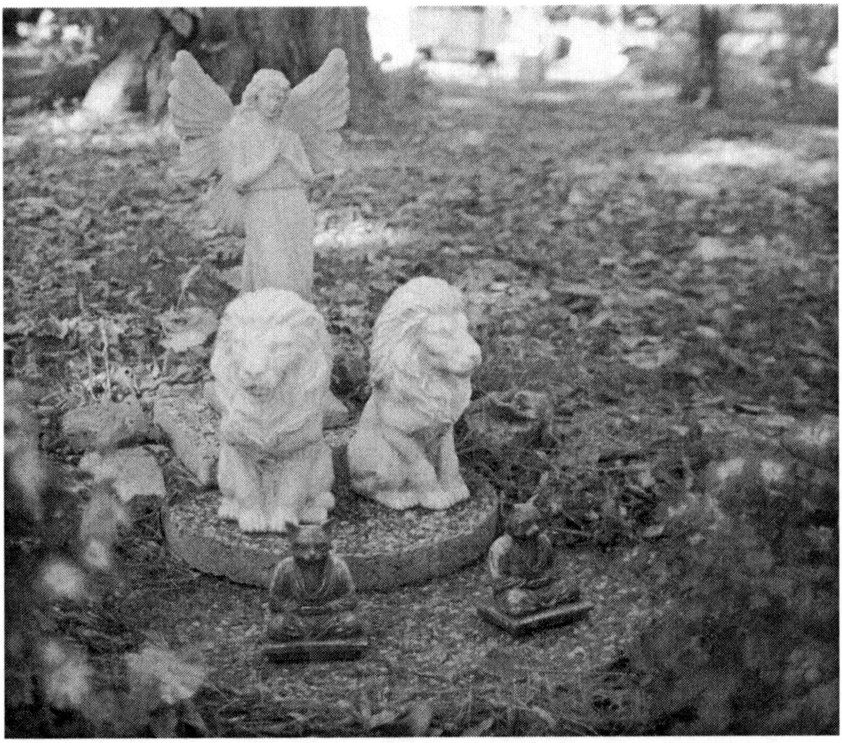

Jac Hapka's gravesite in southern Wisconsin

My search for decorations lasted well into February. Eventually, I found an elegant angel statue, two classic lions, and a pair of cat figurines wearing karate uniforms.

Planning Jac's gravesite proved therapeutic. The pain of his death began to fade, and many years of wonderful memories began to shine through.

I landscaped Jac's grave on a picturesque day in May. This provided me with a much-needed opportunity to honor my friend and gain closure on this chapter of my life.

On the advice of a landscaper, I purchased large decorative patio blocks to create multiple tiers on which the statues would rest. A local gardener suggested chrysanthemums and wildflowers. I was pleased with the outcome, and neighbors often stop to admire Jac's gravesite while passing my parents' home.

FREQUENTLY ASKED QUESTIONS

Thousands of pet owners have written to me, asking questions about FIV. The most commonly asked questions include the following:

Should I vaccinate my FIV+ cat?
Should I spay or neuter my FIV+ cat?
How is FIV spread?
Should I isolate my FIV+ cat?
Can I get AIDS from my FIV+ cat?
Are my dogs and other pets at risk?
Is the FIV vaccine safe?

Should I vaccinate my FIV+ cat?

NO! Cats with FIV should NEVER be vaccinated.

Vaccines contain samples of actual disease organisms. When vaccines work properly, the animal's immune system responds by killing these organisms. This process is supposed to help the immune system develop a defense against the disease contained in the vaccination.

FIV+ cats have impaired immune systems that generally aren't strong enough to fend off the disease organisms contained in vaccines. Furthermore, vaccinations can confuse the immune system, leaving the animal defenseless against disease.

FIV+ cats often become seriously ill after receiving vaccinations. In fact, vaccinations can send an otherwise healthy FIV+ cat into full blown Feline AIDS. I have received heartbreaking emails from pet owners who saw their cats deteriorate or die after receiving vaccinations.

Holistic practitioners often recommend the homeopathic remedy Thuja 30C for cats experiencing adverse reactions to vaccines. One dose, given as soon as possible after the vaccine is administered, can greatly minimize side effects.

Another option is Natramed Vaccine Detox Tabs, available from Feelgood Natural Health (877.677.7797). This combination homeopathic remedy can be used for more serious vaccine reactions. Some practitioners I've consulted recommend 1 to 2 tablets, given twice daily for a period of up to two weeks.

For more information about the potential risks of vaccines, please visit: felineaids.org/vaccinelinks.html .

Should I spay or neuter my FIV+ cat?

Spaying and neutering can help control the feline overpopulation problem. However, precautions must be taken before performing such a procedure on an FIV+ cat.

Many veterinary clinics spay or neuter cats and vaccinate them on the same day. This is a mistake, and the results can be serious.

Vaccinations are a bad idea for any cat with FIV. Administering vaccinations just before or after surgery when the immune system is already compromised is extremely dangerous and places the infected cat at maximum risk. Many cats with FIV have died after undergoing this ill-advised process.

FIV+ cats should never have surgery when they are acutely ill (running a fever, fighting a cold, and so on). Your cat should be as healthy as possible before undergoing any procedure. To further reduce the possibility of FIV related complications, you should increase your cat's dietary nutrition before and after surgery.

How Is FIV spread?

Unlike other feline diseases, FIV is not wildly contagious. A healthy cat cannot get FIV by sitting in the same room with an infected cat. Furthermore, FIV is NOT spread through mutual grooming, shared bedding, food dishes, water bowls, or litter pans.

Some evidence suggests the disease can be passed from mothers to their unborn kittens. However, FIV is primarily spread through deep, penetrating bite wounds. The highest rate of transmission occurs among un-neutered, street-roaming males. These cats get into fights during which they bite each other violently and subsequently spread the disease.

The best way to avoid FIV infection is by keeping your cat out of street fights. If your cat has already been diagnosed with FIV, begin proper treatment immediately (even if the animal isn't showing symptoms).

It should be noted that many kittens test positive for FIV, even when they don't have the disease. Their blood contains antibodies that can trigger erroneous test results. However, if there is any reason to suspect your cat or kitten may have FIV, be proactive and begin treatment immediately.

Should I isolate my FIV+ cat?

Vets often recommend isolating cats infected with FIV. I've encountered nervous pet owners who locked their FIV+ cat in a bedroom, bathroom or basement to prevent their other cats from getting FIV. This separation strategy is misguided, ineffective, and I don't recommend it.

FIV is rarely spread amongst cats living in the same house. The disease is not spread through casual contact, and cats can live together for many years without ever sharing the disease.

You should also consider the emotional impact of separation. If your cats are close or accustomed to spending time together, separation could be traumatic for them.

Jac was extremely close to our other cats, and his absence would have been upsetting to them. Likewise, it would have been stressful for Jac to be separated from the cats he lived with for so long. After weighing the factors involved, I made the decision not to separate Jac from our other cats.

Can I get AIDS from my cat?

NO! It is not possible to get AIDS from your cat.

FIV or Feline AIDS is exclusively a feline disease. It only affects cats. It is impossible for a human to get Feline AIDS.

FIV is not the same disease as the HIV or AIDS that people get. They are completely different diseases.

People often get scared when they learn their cat has Feline AIDS. They hear the word AIDS and panic before getting the facts. Please rest assured that you cannot get AIDS from your cat.

Are my dogs and other pets at risk?

No. Feline AIDS only affects cats. The disease poses no threat to dogs and other animals.

Is the Feline AIDS vaccine safe?

Vaccinations of any kind are dangerous for cats with FIV. Furthermore, the Feline AIDS vaccine is not a cure for the disease, as some people mistakenly believe. There is no therapeutic benefit to this vaccination. It won't cure your FIV+ cat.

A serious consequence of the Feline AIDS vaccination is that it causes cats to test FIV+ indefinitely. If such a cat becomes lost and ends up in an animal shelter, he or she might be euthanized as an FIV+ cat. This is another reason I don't recommend this vaccine.

The vaccine for FIV is still relatively new, and its long-term effects are not yet known. None of my cats will receive this vaccine because I strongly believe there are better ways to protect them from FIV.

USEFUL PRODUCTS AND SERVICES

Vitamins and Supplements

The supplements listed in this section are ones I'm most familiar with. I've thoroughly researched each of these companies and know their products to be of good quality. Keep in mind that you may not find these brands at your local store - products vary from region to region. Fortunately, all of these supplements are available online, and many other good products are available at natural supplement stores.

- **NOW Foods** is an outstanding company that offers a diverse range of quality products at prices lower than many other brands. I often use their products when making the sports drink. They have a new online store, making their products accessible nationwide.

  To order by phone: 1.888.301.1336
  Website: http://www.thecatalog.com

  - Vitamins A and E: NOW Foods sells quality Vitamin A and E supplements at prices that rival those of many discount stores. NOTE: Hundreds of companies make these vitamins, and there are an abundance of possible substitutes.

  - Calcium Ascorbate Powder: This buffered form of vitamin C has no taste or smell, and it generally doesn't cause stomach upset. It's the primary form of vitamin C I use when making the sports drink. The calcium ascorbate powder from NOW Foods is the purest and most affordable product I've found anywhere, but all of the major health food store chains carry their own versions.

- Ester C: This is another buffered form of vitamin C that can be used in the sports drink. NOTE: You don't need multiple forms of vitamin C to make the sports drink. One is sufficient.

- Brewers Yeast: This supplement is a natural source of B-vitamins and amino acids. Many cats like the taste, and it is usually well-tolerated.

- Acidophilus: Medical and holistic vets often recommend acidophilus supplements to help restore the normal balance of bacteria in the colon, especially when antibiotics have been used. This is another important product for cats with FIV.

- L-Lysine: Holistic practitioners often use this amino acid when treating FIV+ cats for upper-respiratory infections, mouth sores, and herpes-related eye problems. NOW Foods offers encapsulated L-Lysine, and a pure powder form that contains no fillers, binders, or preservatives.

- Pycnogenol and CoQ10: Both of these supplements can stimulate a faltering immune system. Holistic practitioners often use them when treating FIV+ cats, especially those afflicted with mouth problems.

- **Animal Essentials** is another good company that makes pure products, including herbal tinctures and nutritional supplements.

  To order by phone: 1.888.463.7748
  Website: www.animalessentials.com

  - Calcium From The Sea: This high-quality supplement, derived from seaweed, provides a rich source of calcium, magnesium, boron, and zinc. NOTE: Now Foods and Only Natural Pet Store offer bone meal and other premium supplements that can also be used as a source of calcium in the sports drink.

- **Orthomolecular Specialties** offers an exceptional line of products that can benefit immune-compromised cats. Their product line was designed by Dr. Wendell O. Belfied, who specializes in nutritional therapies for small animals.

  Website: http://www.belfield.com/

  - Mega C: This potent product contains sodium ascorbate, a form of vitamin C many holistic practitioners believe is most effective in treating cats with immune system disorders. As the name implies, Mega C is highly concentrated – even small doses contain substantial quantities of vitamin C. I often use this supplement as the primary source of vitamin C in the sports drink.

- Beta Plex High B Potency Complex: This B-complex supplement for cats can be used in the sports drink as an alternative to brewers yeast. Beta Plex provides a balanced combination of B-vitamins that help support the immune system.

Combination Homeopathic Remedies

- **Pets 4 Homeopathy**
  Website: http://pets4homeopathy.com

- **Newton Homeopathics**
  Website: www.newtonlabs.net

- **King Bio**
  Website: www.kingbio.com

Single Homeopathic Remedies

- **Washington Homeopathic Products** sells a broad range of single homeopathic remedies. They are open every day and offer express shipping options.

  To order by phone: 1.800.336.1695
  Website: http://homeopathyworks.com

- Pulsatilla 30C: Holistic practitioners often give this remedy to cats with breathing difficulties caused by upper respiratory infections. I've cared for many FIV+ cats who recovered from breathing difficulties while receiving pulsatilla. The remedy is also used for dying pets with loud or labored breathing - it makes breathing easier and helps them get comfortable.

- **Ainsworth Homeopathic Pharmacy** is based in London, England. They offer a broad spectrum of homeopathic remedies and animal nosodes.

  To order by phone: 011.44.7935.5330
  Website: http://www.ainsworths.com

Holistic Practitioners

- **Lita Radford**

  Lita Radford, of pets4homeopathy.com, is a skilled holistic practitioner who specializes in combination homeopathic remedies. She has experience with FIV and several other conditions. I've consulted with her many times. Her consultation fees are the most reasonable I've found, making her services accessible to pet owners on a budget.

  Email: DetoxRules@aol.com

- **Samantha Tobias**

  Samantha Tobias practices in the United Kingdom, and has extensive experience with cats. Her services are reasonably priced and she comes highly recommended by Lita Radford and many pet owners.

  Email: AHH-UK@leahs.freeserve.co.uk

Other Products

- **Aloe Vera Juice**

    - Horse Magic Aloe Vera: Aloe Vera juice can help to relieve digestive disorders and many other health problems. NOTE: Aloe Vera products sold in supermarkets and natural supplement stores often contain preservatives like sodium benzoate and benzoic acid, which are poisonous to cats. Warren Laboratories created the "Horse Magic" product line specifically for pets, and it is free of preservatives.

      To order by phone: 1.800.232.2563
      Website: http://www.warrenlabsaloe.com

- **Laxatives and Digestive Enzymes**

    - Capra Mineral Whey: Made from goat's milk, this powdered supplement contains an abundance of minerals and enzymes. It soothes the intestines and helps to relieve constipation. Many practitioners use this as an alternative to harsh prescription-grade products.

      To order by phone: 1.877.673.0224
      Website: http://www.primaldefense.net/

    - Vetbasis Hairball Remedy: Laxative products sold in veterinary clinics often contain sodium benzoate, which is toxic to cats. Vetbasis Hairball Remedy is petroleum-free and doesn't contain sodium benzoate. This product contains cod liver and vegetable oils, as well as other natural ingredients that lubricate the digestive tract, allowing hairballs and stools to slide through more easily.

To order by phone: 1.703.299.5044
Website: http://www.petsage.com

Natural Supplement Stores

- **Whole Foods** boasts one of America's largest chains of natural supplement stores. They have locations in several states, and they may have stores in your area.

  Corporate office: 1.512.477.4455
  Website: http://www.wholefoodsmarket.com

- **Wild Oats** is another large chain that carries premium quality supplements. Check their website for locations.

  Corporate Office: 1.303.440.5220
  Website: http://www.wildoats.com/

Pet Supply Stores

- **Pet Sage** carries a good selection of combination herbal and homeopathic remedies, premium pet foods, cat toys, and other useful supplies.

  To order by phone: 1.703.299.5044
  Website: http://petsage.com

  - OL Immune: This herbal tincture from Animals Apawthecary contains a blend of olive leaf extract and echinacea, intended to support the immune system and fight infection. It has been formulated to reduce the risk of choking or stomach upset often caused by herbal tinctures.

- **Pets Naturally** carries a vast selection of products, including herbal and homeopathic remedies, as well as nutritional supplements. They also stock the Animal Essentials product line and a number of premium pet foods. Their staff is highly knowledgeable, and I've come to regard this store as an invaluable resource.

  To order by phone: 1.818.784.1233

- **Only Natural Pet Store** is an online pet supply store with a diverse inventory that includes a broad spectrum of herbal and homeopathic products. They also stock an excellent selection of nutritional supplements, including the Vetri-Science product line. I would encourage anyone caring for an FIV+ cat to visit this online store.

  To order by phone: 1.888.937.6677
  Website: www.onlynaturalpet.com

  - Vetri-Science Cardio Strength: This unique supplement has been designed to support cardiovascular function in elderly and ailing cats. It contains CoQ10, as well as the amino acids L-Taurine and L-Carnitine, supplements often prescribed by holistic practitioners when caring for cats with serious heart conditions.

- Pet Immune Balance: This product contains plant-derived sterols and sterolins, which have shown promise in the treatment of FIV. These potent natural substances can calm an overactive immune system or boost one that is weak.

- Solid Gold Berry Balance: This premium product has been formulated to support healthy urinary tract function. It contains cranberry extract, vitamin C, and other natural ingredients that have proven helpful in fighting urinary tract infections and dissolving urinary crystals.
  NOTE: NaturVet (www.naturvet.com) also makes an excellent cranberry formula called Cranberry Relief. For homeopathic treatment of bladder infections, Natural Pet Pharmaceuticals (http://natural-pet.com/) makes an effective combination remedy called Urinary Tract Irritations. I have used the above-referenced products in combination while caring for my own cats who were battling stubborn urinary tract infections.

ABOUT THE AUTHOR

Thomas Hapka is a freelance writer and graduate of the University of Wisconsin-Whitewater. He learned of FIV in 1995 when his cat, Jac, was diagnosed. Since then, he has consulted with hundreds of pet owners. His clients have spanned nine countries and included two American zoos. Hapka has been featured in the magazines Australian National Cat and Cat's Life. His web site, felineaids.org, has received more than 80,000 visitors.

---

[1] Price-Pottenger Nutrition Foundation, *Pottenger's Cats – A Study In Nutrition*, (2000).
Available at http://price-pottenger.org/Articles/PottsCats.htm
(24 February 2004).

[2] Alternative Medicine, *How Homeopathy Works*, (2004).
Available at http://www.alternativemedicine.com/
(18 February 2004).

[3] Greenbrier Veterinary Hospital, *Feline Leukemia Virus Diseases*, (2004). Available at http://greenbriervet.com/newsletters/felv.htm
(12 February 2004)

[4] Moore Veterinary Hospital, *Feline Infectious Peritonitis*, (2004).
Available at http://moorevet.com/Feline/FIP.html
(15 February 2004)

[5] Vitamin World, *What is Vitamin C?*, (2003). Available at
http://vitamin-world.org/vitamins/15/Vitamin-C
(14 February 2004)